ACTION PLAN FOR
OSTEOPOROSIS

KERRI WINTERS-STONE, PHD

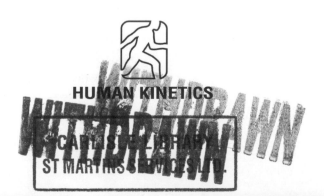

HUMAN KINETICS

Library of Congress Cataloging-in-Publication Data

Winters-Stone, Kerri, 1969-
  Action plan for osteoporosis / Kerri Winters-Stone.
    p. cm.
  Includes bibliographical references and index.
  ISBN 0-7360-5482-0 (soft cover)
  1. Osteoporosis–Popular works. I. Title.
  RC931.073W598 2005
  616.7'16–dc22

                          2004030253

ISBN: 0-7360-5482-0

Acquisitions Editor: Martin Barnard; **Developmental Editor:** Leigh Keylock; **Assistant Editor:** Carla Zych; **Copyeditor:** Barbara Field; **Proofreader:** Sue Fetters; **Indexer:** Betty Frizzéll; **Permission Manager:** Carly Breeding; **Graphic Designer:** Fred Starbird; **Graphic Artist:** Sandra Meier; **Photo Manager:** Dan Wendt; **Cover Designer:** Jack W. Davis; **Photographer (interior):** Dan Wendt, unless otherwise noted; **Art Manager and Illustrator:** Kareema McLendon; **Printer:** United Graphics

ACSM Publications Committee Chair: Jeffery L. Roitman, EdD, FACSM; **ACSM Communications and Public Information Committee Chair:** Harold W. Kohl, PhD, FACSM; **ACSM Group Publisher:** D. Mark Robertson; **ACSM Editorial Manager:** Lori A. Tish

Human Kinetics books are available at special discounts for bulk purchase. Special editions or book excerpts can also be created to specification. For details, contact the Special Sales Manager at Human Kinetics.

Printed in the United States of America   10 9 8 7 6 5 4 3 2 1

Human Kinetics
Web site: www.HumanKinetics.com

United States: Human Kinetics
P.O. Box 5076, Champaign, IL 61825-5076
800-747-4457
e-mail: humank@hkusa.com

Canada: Human Kinetics
475 Devonshire Road Unit 100
Windsor, ON N8Y 2L5
800-465-7301 (in Canada only)
e-mail: orders@hkcanada.com

Europe: Human Kinetics
107 Bradford Road, Stanningley
Leeds LS28 6AT, United Kingdom
+44 (0) 113 255 5665
e-mail: hk@hkeurope.com

Australia: Human Kinetics
57A Price Avenue
Lower Mitcham, South Australia 5062
08 8277 1555
e-mail: liaw@hkaustralia.com

New Zealand: Human Kinetics
Division of Sports Distributors NZ Ltd.
P.O. Box 300 226 Albany
North Shore City, Auckland
0064 9 448 1207
e-mail: blairc@hknewz.com

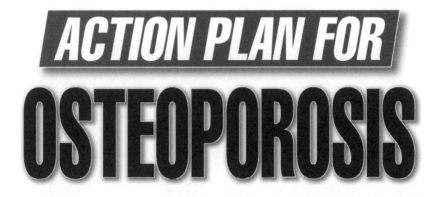

ACTION PLAN FOR
OSTEOPOROSIS

CONTENTS

INTRODUCTION

Osteoporosis is a disease characterized by low bone mass and poor bone structure that develops over time and leads to increased risk of fracture. Osteoporosis is also known as "porous bone disease," "brittle bone disease," or the "silent disease." You are most likely reading this book because you or someone you know has osteoporosis or is at risk for developing it and you are looking for answers on how to battle this disease. This brief introduction is intended to improve your understanding of the prevalence and impact of osteoporosis and particularly to clear up any common misconceptions about this disease. In chapter 1, we will explore the development and detection of osteoporosis in greater detail, and the remaining chapters will discuss how you can improve your bone and muscle health so that you can lower your risk of fracture. Most of the book will focus on how exercise can lower your fracture risk, but we will also talk about nutritional strategies and medications aimed at bone health.

Osteoporosis is not uncommon.   Osteoporosis is a reality or a threat for more than 55 percent of Americans over the age of 50 (National Osteoporosis Foundation 2004). Nearly 10 million American women and men already have osteoporosis and another 34 million are at risk for developing the disease because they have below-normal bone mass (osteopenia) (Looker et al. 1997). Nearly one in two women and one in four men over 50 will experience an osteoporosis-related fracture in their lifetime. A woman's risk of fracturing a hip is equal to her combined risk of developing breast, uterine, and ovarian cancer.

The number of people with osteoporosis is projected to grow as our society expands and ages, so if you have osteoporosis or low bone mass, clearly you aren't alone. In response to the growing number of people with osteoporosis, research on osteoporosis treatment and prevention has escalated over the past 20 years. This book will provide you with the most up-to-date information on how to best reduce your risk of fracture based on the latest evidence from research. Thus, you can be assured that the information presented here is scientifically tested and sound.

Osteoporosis can strike at any age.   Osteoporosis is more likely to be diagnosed in older people because the disease develops over time and bone mass is lost as we age. In women, bone loss speeds up for a short time after menopause, and in some women this can lead to significant bone loss by age 60. Since men do not go through menopause, they tend to get osteoporosis at a later age, usually between 70 and 80, but certain medications or conditions can lead to an increased risk of osteoporosis at an earlier age in men.

Some people are more likely to have below-average bone mass at any point in their life because of genetics. In such individuals, the presence or onset of risk factors that cause bone to be lost more quickly or sooner than normally expected could lead to early development of osteoporosis. Circumstances that could lead to early bone loss are shown in the following sidebar.

Possible Causes of Early Bone Loss

► Natural, surgical (hysterectomy), or chemical (drug-induced) menopause before the age of 45

► Irregular or absent menstrual cycles before menopause

► Anorexia nervosa

► Any condition that decreases testosterone levels in men (surgical removal of testes, anti-testosterone drugs)

► Long-term use or high doses of corticosteroids (e.g., prednisone) or anti-seizure medications

► A significant decrease in or low physical activity

► A significant decrease in calcium or vitamin D intake or availability

► Certain medical conditions

Osteoporosis can strike men.   Once thought of only as a women's disease, osteoporosis is now known to occur in men as well. Since we are living longer and are better at evaluating bone health, a growing number of men are now found to have or to be at risk for osteoporosis. Women are more likely to have osteoporosis than men and are younger when the disease develops; however, nearly one in five people with osteoporosis and one in three people with low bone mass are men (Looker et al. 1997). Twenty-five percent of men over 50 will suffer an osteoporosis-related fracture in their lifetime, and men tend to have poorer outcomes from a fracture than women. Most risk factors for osteoporosis are the same for men and women (see chapter 1). The information in this book can help both women and men reduce their risk of fracture.

Osteoporosis does not discriminate.   Although Caucasians and Asians have a higher rate of osteoporosis than other racial and ethnic groups, people of all backgrounds can be at risk for the disease (National Osteoporosis

Foundation 2004). About 10 percent of Hispanic women have osteoporosis and another 49 percent are at risk because they have low bone mass. About 1 in 20 African American women have osteoporosis and 35 percent are at risk. Racial and ethnic differences in bone health are mostly attributable to genetic differences in bone mass. For example, African Americans tend to have stronger bones throughout their life span, so age- and menopause-related bone loss are better tolerated. The risk factors for osteoporosis (except race) and for bone loss are similar for all people regardless of race and ethnicity. Individuals of all backgrounds should be aware of their risk factors for osteoporosis and take steps to optimize their bone health. Although specific research on the topic is scarce, the effectiveness of osteoporosis treatment and prevention strategies in offsetting bone loss should not differ among racial and ethnic groups.

Osteoporosis has many causes.   Osteoporosis is rarely attributed to a single cause and is more often the result of several factors working together to lower bone mass. The risk factors that contribute to osteoporosis are listed in detail in chapter 1. What causes bone loss and osteoporosis for one individual may not be the same for another. The presence of multiple risk factors may indicate a greater risk for disease. For example, a 65-year-old woman is at higher risk for osteoporosis than a 65-year-old man because she has twice as many risk factors for osteoporosis as he does. They are both at risk because of their age, but because women usually have lower bone mass due to their smaller size and lose bone during menopause, she is at higher risk.

Since osteoporosis and bone loss can be caused by many factors acting together, knowing which and how many risk factors you have will help in determining whether bone loss is a health concern for you. Because many fractures are the result of both osteoporosis and falls, knowing your risk factors for falls is also important. A risk factor assessment is usually conducted as part of an osteoporosis evaluation since this information will help guide treatment decisions. Chapter 2 lists factors that can help determine your risk of falling. A prudent approach to lowering fracture risk is to address the underlying risks and causes of bone loss as well as fall risk. Because physical activity is known to slow or prevent bone loss, as well as to prevent falls, the exercises outlined in this book may be part of a targeted plan to keep your bones together!

Osteoporosis can progress without pain.   Osteoporosis is also called the "silent disease" because bone loss does not result in any noticeable symptoms, such as pain. In fact, if you never suffered a fracture, you could live your whole life with osteoporosis without ever knowing it. Fractures that result from osteoporosis, however, often cause considerable pain. If someone is experiencing pain near a joint or in a limb but does not have a fracture, the pain is more likely related to a muscle or connective tissue (ligaments and tendons) problem. The fact that bone loss can go unnoticed underscores the importance of knowing your risk factors for osteoporosis and having your bone health evaluated when risk factors are present.

Osteoporosis can be lived with.   People with osteoporosis are not doomed to have a fracture. True osteoporotic fractures are those in which the bone cannot withstand the weight of the body and simply collapses. Such fractures are relatively rare, and it is more likely that some type of low force trauma (e.g., a fall, a sudden twisting movement, violent coughing or sneezing, improper lifting) causes an already weakened bone to break. With proper treatment of bone loss and adoption of strategies that reduce fracture risk, such as exercise, someone could live a lifetime with osteoporosis and never suffer a fracture.

Osteoporosis can be treated.   There is no cure for osteoporosis, but several prescription medications are available that increase or maintain bone mass and reduce fracture risk. Chapter 9 presents an overview of these treatments. Proper nutrition and targeted exercise are also important complements to medication in promoting overall health and lowering the risk of falls.

Osteoporosis-related fractures can be prevented.   As discussed earlier, fractures are not inevitable if you have osteoporosis or are at risk for developing it. Although some fractures are simply unavoidable (such as breaking an arm after slipping on ice), several strategies can be employed to decrease the likelihood of breaking a bone. We know that the use of certain prescription medications reduces the likelihood of fractures by increasing bone mass (see chapter 9). We know that adequate calcium and vitamin D intake are important for slowing bone loss and perhaps even preventing falls (see chapter 8). We know that making your home environment safer can reduce the risk of falling (see chapter 2). Although exercise has not been clinically tested for its ability to reduce fractures per se, we know that it can build bone mass or slow bone loss and that it has been clinically proven to decrease the occurrence of falls. Both of these strategies are central to reducing fracture risk. The focus of this book is to teach you how to exercise to strengthen your bones and muscles so that you can maximize your ability to lower your risk of fracture.

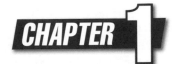

CHAPTER 1

THRIVING WITH OSTEOPOROSIS

To better understand osteoporosis, you need to understand the skeleton itself and how mineral loss from the skeleton can lead to osteoporosis. Armed with this knowledge, you'll be able to understand how your behaviors and choices can affect the health of your bones either positively or negatively.

For most of us, when we think about the skeleton, images of Halloween characters and anatomy class come to mind. Skeletons never seem to be alive, unless there's a cute little six-year-old wriggling inside her holiday costume. We have a hard time comprehending that the skeleton is actually a living organ that is constantly undergoing change in response to both internal and external influences. At our laboratory, when we show patients the image created by a test that gives us a picture of their skeleton, most exclaim, "Wow, that's me? How *weird.*" Although we don't really feel that our bones are alive until we break them, we must keep in mind that bones are made of living, changing tissue that needs just as much TLC as our heart, brain, lungs, and muscles to keep our entire body strong.

The skeleton serves many important purposes in the body. The one we most commonly think of is that it provides a framework for the body. The skeleton is what we "hang" our muscles on and what allows us to stand upright and move about in our environment. Thus, the skeleton must be strong enough not only to support our body weight but also to allow us to play hard, to exercise vigorously, and to withstand injuries in unfortunate cases such as falling onto hard ground. The skeleton must be able to tolerate all of this without breaking. You can quickly see how a weakened skeleton could break more easily. But as important as this function of the skeleton is, the bones play several other critical roles in the body.

The skeleton also protects vital organs such as the brain and heart from trauma. The inner cavities of some bones help make new red blood cells. And a particularly important function of the skeleton is to serve as a reservoir for calcium; more than 99 percent of the calcium in the body is stored in the skeleton. Virtually all of this calcium is in the form of bone crystals that give bone its hardness and its strength. But this skeletal warehouse of calcium is also a pool of mineral that can be readily called upon when blood levels of calcium become low. We need calcium in our blood for functions such as nerve transmission, blood clotting, hormone actions, and many more. Calcium is an essential nutrient, meaning that we must derive it from our diet because we cannot make it in our bodies. Thus, when we aren't getting enough calcium in our diet to keep our blood levels normal, calcium is borrowed from the reservoir in the skeleton. Again, it's easy to see how a diet low in calcium can cause the skeleton to be robbed of the calcium supply that gives it strength. We'll talk more about nutrition in chapter 8.

Pursuing Bone Balance

For bone to accomplish many of the tasks we discussed, it must be able to change and keep itself functioning properly. The skeleton must be able to keep itself strong by adding new bone to places that need it and take it away form places that don't. Bone is in a state of constant turnover where some bone cells are breaking down old and weak bone while other bone cells are building new, strong bone. In an adult skeleton, the processes of breaking down and building bone normally occur at similar rates, and bone balance is typical over the period of middle adulthood (18 to 50 years of age); however, when either or both of these processes are altered, an imbalance occurs and bone is either lost or gained.

Many different processes can upset bone balance (see figure 1.1). With age, bone breakdown outpaces buildup, causing us to lose up to 1 percent of our bone per year after age 30 (Hui et al. 1999). Certain conditions, such as estrogen loss from menopause or an overactive thyroid gland, may increase bone breakdown and slow down bone buildup, causing further bone loss (Riggs 2002). On the other hand, pharmaceutical agents that stop the breakdown of bone or physical activity that causes bone to build up can cause a gain of bone. In the growing skeleton, bone balance is also disrupted, but at this stage bone building far exceeds bone breakdown, causing the skeleton to grow in length and strength. Some have suggested the growing period (from ages 3 to 18 years) is the best time to improve bone health through better nutrition and more activity (Fuchs et al. 2001; McKay et al. 2000). However, since bone is a dynamic tissue throughout life, strategies to slow down the breakdown of bone and to build new, stronger bone are useful at any life stage. We must also

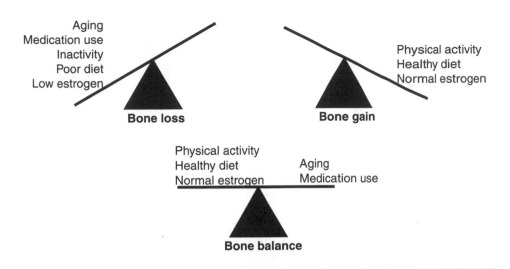

Figure 1.1   The balance among factors that determine bone health at any point in life. The middle scale illustrates a situation in which the factors are equal, resulting in bone balance and no change in bone mass. In the scale on the left, negative factors outweigh positive ones and bone mass is lost. In the scale on the right, positive factors outweigh negative ones and bone is gained.

keep in mind, though, that many factors influence the state of our bones at any given time. This book will teach you how exercising your bones can keep them healthy and will also help you better understand all the factors that influence your risk for osteoporosis so you can make the best choices for your bones!

Defining Osteoporosis

Osteoporosis is a condition characterized by low bone mass and poor bone structure that in combination lead to an increased risk of fractures. In figure 1.2, you can see how the osteoporotic bone at the top has less mass and fewer connections compared to the healthy bone at the bottom. Osteoporotic bone is like a building that is being eaten away by termites. When the termites eat the wood, they are eating away at the infrastructure of the house. If an event were to occur that would test the house's ability to stand, such as a tree branch falling on it or a small earthquake, it would likely collapse. Likewise, if the termites were so numerous and so hungry that they ate right through the support beams, the house would fold like a deck of cards without any help from Mother Nature. Just as wood being eaten away from a house makes it more likely to fall apart, losing bone mass puts our bones at greater risk for collapse.

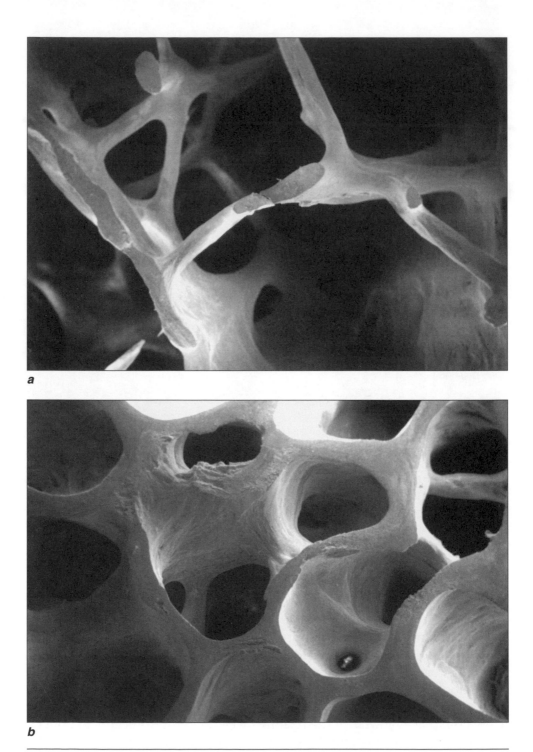

a

b

Figure 1.2 In these microscopic photos, the osteoporotic bone *(a)* is thinner and less connected than the healthy bone *(b)*.

Reproduced from *J Bone Miner Res* 1986: 1: 15-21, with permission of the American Society for Bone and Mineral Research.

Osteoporosis can occur at any age but is most prevalent past the age of 50 and is thus considered an age-related disease. As with most chronic diseases, osteoporosis does not develop overnight but rather over a lifetime.

Our bones are growing most rapidly in length and strength during childhood and adolescence. After they finish growing in length, our bones change very little until we reach the age of 30. After 30, our bones gradually lose mineral throughout our lifetime, and although the actual loss per year is rather small (1 percent), this can add up to a substantial loss by the time we are in our 50s (see figure 1.3). In addition, certain diseases or conditions may accelerate bone loss over discrete time periods. For example, when a woman reaches menopause and estrogen levels decrease, bone loss increases. During the first five years after menopause, bone loss can increase two to five times but then tends to slow to normal rates of loss thereafter. Because of the progressive nature of the disease, it is difficult to tell that it is developing. Since bone loss is not painful, someone who is experiencing it may not know it is happening until a fracture occurs. Luckily, we have effective methods of detecting osteoporosis and bone loss before that happens, and we'll talk more about them later. But the bottom line is that any time is the right time to make good choices for bone health. By doing so, you can decrease your risk of osteoporosis and fractures or reduce the severity of your osteoporosis if you already have it (figure 1.3).

Osteoporosis is a clinical condition that puts one at greater risk of fracture from what otherwise should be tolerable loads. In other words, we should be able to pick up our groceries, sneeze, twist rapidly (as in golfing), or even fall accidentally without an injury, save a possible strain or bruise. With osteoporosis, these types of events may put enough stress on the bones to cause them to fracture. Falling is the most typical event

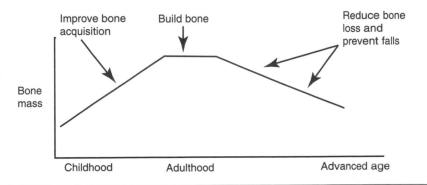

Figure 1.3 The theoretical change in bone mass throughout the life span and how interventions that either slow bone loss or increase bone mass affect it.
Adapted, by permission, from C.M. Snow, J.M. Shaw, K.M. Winters and K.A Witzke, 2003, "Bone health across the lifespan—exercising our options," *Exercise and Sport Sciences Review* 31(3): 117-122.

associated with a fracture, so we'll talk about falling at length in later chapters and discuss specific exercises that can reduce the risk of falling. What must be realized, though, is that osteoporosis is not an "either-or" condition. In other words, one's bone health, and thus degree of fracture risk, is on a continuum (see figure 1.4). As the disease progresses from mild to moderate to severe, the risk of fracture increases. It is similar to heart disease in that as the number of blocked arteries increases, the risk of a heart attack becomes successively greater. Likewise, our bone health lies on a continuum so that we can predict our risk of getting osteoporosis before the disease occurs. A special test (which we'll discuss later in this chapter) can tell us if we have osteoporosis, osteopenia (low bone mass), or normal bones. Some of you may already know your risk for osteoporosis.

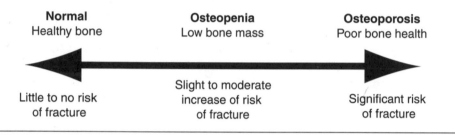

Figure 1.4 The continuum of bone health.

Understanding the Development of Osteoporosis

The development of osteoporosis is complex, and no single factor is solely to blame for the disease. Some of the factors can be controlled and others cannot (table 1.1). Uncontrollable factors that influence bone health include genetics, gender, race, age, and bone loss secondary to disease. Genetics have already predetermined up to two-thirds of our bone mass. A family history of osteoporosis, particularly with related fractures, is a significant risk factor for future disease. Women are at higher risk for osteoporosis due to their smaller frame and vulnerability to estrogen-related bone loss following menopause. But approximately 20 percent of osteoporosis cases occur in men, and this percentage may increase as men live longer and awareness of disease risk in men increases. Osteoporosis is more prevalent among Caucasian and Asian women compared to African American and Hispanic women, although a recent report suggests hip fracture rates are on the rise among Hispanic women in California (Zingmond et al. 2004). Disease prevalence in other races has not been well described. Racial differences may be attributable to differences in bone size, muscle mass, or dietary calcium. Aging accounts for slow bone loss and begins as we approach our thirties (Riggs et al. 1986). Over time, this gradual but consistent loss of bone can lead to

Table 1.1   Selected Risk Factors for Osteoporosis

Risk factors you cannot control
• Being female
• Being thin or having a small frame
• Advanced age
• A family history of osteoporosis
• Being postmenopausal, including early or surgically induced menopause
• Low testosterone levels in men
• Being Caucasian or Asian, although African Americans and Hispanic Americans may be at risk as well
Risk factors you can control
• A diet low in calcium
• An inactive lifestyle
• Cigarette smoking
• Excessive use of alcohol
Risk factors you may be able to control
• Abnormal absence of menstrual periods (amenorrhea)
• Anorexia nervosa
• Use of certain medications, such as corticosteroids and anticonvulsants

greater risk of fracture. Thus, osteoporosis is most often diagnosed after the age of 50, except in infrequent cases where another disease may be responsible for excessive and early loss of bone. Obviously, we cannot change our genes, gender, race, or age, but we do have control over other influences on our bone health.

Controllable factors that affect bone health include reproductive hormone levels, dietary adequacy (namely, calcium and vitamin D), and physical activity. Near or at the onset of menopause, typically around age 50, women's bodies lose the ability to produce normal levels of estrogen, and this loss of estrogen can cause bone to be lost two to five times more quickly than loss caused by age alone (Gallagher et al. 1987). Estrogen and hormone replacement therapy (HRT), a combination of estrogen and progesterone, has been shown to be effective in stopping menopause-related bone loss (Cummings et al. 2002). Despite this finding, many women are now choosing not to go on HRT because of recent reports that HRT is associated with a slight increase in risk for stroke and breast cancer. Current studies are evaluating whether very low dose estrogen can effectively preserve bone without increasing the risk of stroke or cancer. Whether testosterone plays a similar role to estrogen in male osteoporosis is unclear. Adequate testosterone in men may be necessary to help produce small amounts of estrogen important for bone health. Although some osteoporotic men also have low testosterone levels, low testosterone does not inevitably lead to osteoporosis. Most of the options for maintaining normal hormone levels are drug-related and will be discussed in chapter 9, but other behaviors that help prevent changes in hormone levels include the avoidance of intense exercise training combined with strict dieting. In particular, women who exercise excessively and restrict their eating are prone to disturbances in their menstrual cycle and low estrogen levels. Rest assured that the amount and type of exercise recommended in this book will not put you at risk for such problems.

As discussed earlier, most of the calcium in the body is stored in the bones. We must maintain a steady level of calcium in our body by consuming calcium contained in foods. If our dietary intake of calcium is chronically inadequate, bone will be lost from the skeleton and it will weaken. We also need enough vitamin D in our diet to help get calcium from our stomach into our bloodstream, from which some of that calcium will then go to our bones. Vitamin D may also be important for maintaining strong muscles. Much of our vitamin D is obtained from sun exposure and from fortified dairy foods. Other nutrients that may influence bone health include protein, sodium, and vitamins C and K. Chapter 8 includes a more detailed discussion of how to eat for healthy bones. Adherence to a sensible diet helps keep bones strong by minimizing bone loss that may be due to poor intakes of calcium and vitamin D.

Both gravity and physical movement, or exercise, play an important role in keeping our bones strong. The first evidence of this fact was that people who traveled into space or were immobilized for long periods suffered rapid and dramatic bone loss (Baldwin et al. 1996). Studies have shown that inactive women have lower bone mass than physically active women (Fehling et al. 1995; Robinson et al. 1995) and that physically active people experience fewer fractures even if they have osteoporosis (Gregg et al. 2000). Studies have also shown that when people engage in a certain type and amount of exercise, their rate of bone loss slows; in some cases exercisers even gain bone. Getting moving is definitely something we can control! We will discuss the what, why, where, and how of exercise throughout the rest of this book.

Diagnosing Osteoporosis

It wasn't until the last 20 years that we could precisely determine someone's risk of fracture *before* a fracture actually occurred! Osteoporosis was commonly diagnosed only after a fracture occurred and the person's bones looked practically transparent on an x-ray. With technological advances, we can now assess how strong or weak someone's bones are before they develop osteoporosis and can predict how bone mass may change in response to a change in a lifestyle element such as diet. If someone already has osteoporosis, we can determine the severity of the disease and the effectiveness of interventions such as exercise or medication in reducing the severity.

The gold-standard technique for osteoporosis evaluation is called dual-energy x-ray absorptiometry (DXA). You may also have heard this test called a *bone density test* because it measures *bone mineral density*. Bone density tells us how much hard mineral you have in a given bone, such as the spine or hip. Studies show that bone density is an accurate index of bone strength. The higher your bone density, the stronger your bones are and the less likely they are to fracture. On the other hand, less dense

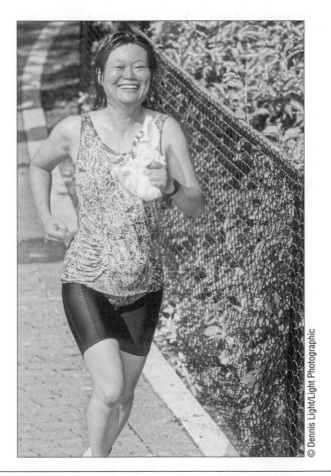

© Dennis Light/Light Photographic

It's never too early to start employing bone-healthy practices such as moderate-intensity weight-bearing exercise.

bones are weaker and more likely to fracture. Thus, a bone density test can give you the best estimate of your *fracture risk*. Bone density is typically measured at the bones that are most often fractured: the hip, spine, and forearm. Bones other than these three may also be at risk of fracture but are harder to measure. Bone density at any of the three measurable sites is a good indicator of the fracture risk of other bones.

Your risk of fracture is evaluated by comparing your bone density values to both age-matched and young-normal reference groups. Age-matched comparisons, also called Z-scores, describe your bone density value relative to others of similar gender, age, and race/ethnicity. The Z-scores are usually translated to a percent score that tells you if you are above or below age-matched norms. For example, if your age-matched score is 120 percent, it means that your bone density is 20 percent above the average bone density for similar women. Likewise, if your bone density is 100 percent, it is equal to that of your peers, and if it is 80 percent, it is 20 percent lower than that of your peers. Although a Z-score can help you see how you compare to others, it does not necessarily tell you about your risk of osteoporosis. Because bone loss is part of the aging process, we can be average for our age but be at risk for or have osteoporosis.

The diagnosis of osteoporosis was established in 1994 by the World Health Organization. It is based on comparison of an individual's bone density to the bone density of a young adult and is called a T-score. T-scores compare an individual's bone density reading with that of an average 25- to 30-year-old of similar gender and race/ethnicity. A T-score equal to or more than 2.5 units below young-normal indicates osteoporosis; a T-score between 1 and 2.5 units below young-normal indicates osteopenia (*low bone mass*); and a T-score less than 1 unit below young-normal ($\geq$-1 SD) indicates absence of disease and is considered normal.

You may have seen advertisements for other types of bone density evaluation tests in your local drugstore or shopping center. These tests are becoming increasingly popular because they can be done in almost any setting, are less expensive than DXA, and emit extremely low or no radiation. However, the *only* test that can diagnose your risk of osteoporosis is a DXA test. The other "bone density tests" should only be regarded as screening tools that may indicate the need to be seen for further testing. The two most popular of such tests are a peripheral DXA, or pDXA, which measures the bone density of the finger, and a heel ultrasound, which estimates the bone density of the heel. Neither of these tests measures bone density at the sites where fractures are most likely to occur, making it difficult to gauge the risk of a hip, spine, or wrist fracture. Furthermore, these tests are not very reliable, and your results may vary as much as 5 to 10 percent on any given day. This could mean that you would be considered normal on one day and osteopenic on another day.

To get the most accurate and reliable measurement of your bone health, ask your physician to perform a DXA bone density test. If your

Bone Density Test Recommendations

A bone density test is recommended for the following individuals/ circumstances (National Osteoporosis Foundation 2004):

▸ All postmenopausal women under age 65 who have one or more additional risk factors for osteoporosis (in addition to being postmenopausal and female; see table 1.1)

▸ All women age 65 and older regardless of additional risk factors

▸ Postmenopausal women with one or more fractures (to confirm diagnosis and determine disease severity)

▸ Women who are considering therapy for osteoporosis if bone density testing would facilitate the decision

▸ Men or women with one or more of the following: prolonged exposure to certain medications, such as steroids used to treat asthma or arthritis, anticonvulsants, and certain cancer treatments; chronic disease that affects the kidneys, lungs, stomach, and intestines and alters hormone levels; or low levels of the sex hormone testosterone

In addition, pre- or perimenopausal women, particularly those with a family history of osteoporosis and more than one risk factor, may wish to have a bone density determination; however, insurance often does not cover the cost of a bone density test for premenopausal women. Early evaluation of bone density, though, could offer the best strategy for preventing age-related declines in bone mass and delaying or offsetting the onset of osteoporosis.

bone density is normal, you may not need to have another test for 5 to 10 years unless you experience a change in the interim that might affect your bone health, such as menopause. If you have osteopenia, your physician may recommend lifestyle modifications such as adjustments in diet and exercise with follow-up testing in one to two years to reassess your bone health. If you have osteoporosis, chances are your physician will recommend some type of drug therapy with follow-up testing in one year to determine the effectiveness of the medication. You may already have had a bone density test and been told that you have osteoporosis or osteopenia. Knowing your bone health will help you use this book most effectively to choose exercises that decrease your risk of fracture or modify your current exercise program to include fracture-risk-reduction exercises. You may also be able to see whether your bone density remains stable or even increases if you have another bone density test after a year of regular exercise.

Summary

The skeleton is a dynamic, changing organ that serves many purposes in the body. The skeleton must manage itself so that it can perform all of the tasks required of it and still remain strong enough to endure all sorts of insults without breaking. The skeleton can keep itself healthy by getting rid of old and weak bone and replacing it with new, strong bone. But factors such as age, poor nutrition, or inactivity can disrupt these processes and result in bone loss. If this disruption is severe or lengthy enough, osteoporosis may result.

Osteoporosis is referred to as the "silent disease" because bone loss is not painful and produces no noticeable symptoms. In the past, the first sign of disease was a fracture, and some fractures were never detected. With the development of new testing methods, such as DXA (*a.k.a.,* bone density test), we can now determine the severity of osteoporosis as well as an individual's risk of getting the disease before it develops. The bone density test tells us how our bones compare to others our age, but most important, it can tell us if we have or are at risk for osteoporosis. Certain guidelines recommend who should have a bone density test, but knowing your bone density is helpful at any age, particularly if you have one or more risk factors for the disease. Bone density can be categorized as normal, osteopenic, or osteoporotic. Depending on the diagnosis, therapy and follow-up testing may be recommended. Exercise may be a recommended therapy, either alone or in addition to medication management. Some of you may already be active, and we will tell you how you can remain active safely and effectively.

ACTION PLAN:
THRIVING WITH OSTEOPOROSIS

- ☐ Understand the definition of osteoporosis.
- ☐ Know which risk factors for osteoporosis you have.
- ☐ Consider an action plan for improving modifiable risk factors.
- ☐ Depending on your risk factors, consider having a DXA bone density test.
- ☐ Become familiar with the concept of T- and Z-scores so that you can best understand the medical interpretation of your bone density test.
- ☐ Understand that screening tools, such as a finger or heel bone density test, are not diagnostic. If either of these tests shows you are at risk for poor bone health, strongly consider having a DXA test performed.

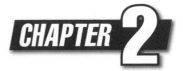
FINDING WAYS TO PREVENT FALLS

As you learned in chapter 1, if you have osteoporosis, you stand a greater risk of fracture. Having osteoporosis does not mean that you will inevitably suffer a fracture, however, nor does having normal or osteopenic bone density mean that you are completely risk free. Some people can live a lifetime with osteoporosis and never fracture, whereas others will never develop severe disease but may break a bone. Although bone density is a strong indicator of fracture risk, we also know that falling may be an equally important risk factor for fracture.

Most fractures in older adults are associated with a fall. About 35 percent of people over age 65 and living in the community fall, and about 25 percent of all falls result in serious injury such as fracture (Cumming 1998; Hornbrook et al. 1994). People who have a combination of osteoporosis and a likelihood of falling are at the greatest risk of fracture, whereas people who have osteoporosis but rarely fall or who have strong bones but fall a lot are less likely to fracture. Factors that increase the likelihood of falling can vary considerably from one person to another. Falls can be the result of a single cause, such as slipping on an icy sidewalk, or more likely the result of many factors working in combination, such as tripping over a phone cord in a dark room and being too weak to stop the fall. Thus, you should be aware of all the possible risk factors for falling and consider those that are most relevant to you when creating a plan to prevent falls.

An accidental fall is one where you suddenly and unintentionally change your position, causing you to land at a lower level, on an object, the floor, or the ground, other than as a consequence of sudden onset of paralysis, epileptic seizure, or overwhelming external force (Tinetti and Williams 1997). For example, by our definition, stumbling on the corner of a coffee table and landing on the carpet would be considered an accidental fall, whereas tumbling onto your knee when a hurried shopper knocks you over trying to get to the sales rack would not.

Recognizing the Causes of Falls

Falls are generally attributable to unsafe environments, the effects of medical conditions and their treatments, or physical declines (see the sidebar below). Such factors can make it more likely for people to lose their balance or footing and fall and also more likely that they will be unable to stop the fall once it has begun. Loss of balance underlies most beginnings of a fall, whereas poor reaction time and muscle weakness underlie the inability to stop a fall. Falling should be a primary concern for all people over age 50 and particularly for those who are elderly or those with osteoporosis or osteopenia. The good news is that many of the factors that contribute to falls can be corrected and many falls can be prevented. In this chapter, I'll describe strategies for fall prevention, and in chapter 6, I'll outline a specific exercise program targeted at preventing falls. Since falls are often caused by multiple factors, the best prevention programs are often a combination of appropriate prevention strategies. The Personal Fall Risk Inventory on page 18 can help you identify which fall risk factors you have and, in turn, which areas you should focus on to reduce your risk of falling.

Risk Factors for Falls

- ▸ Older age
- ▸ Muscle weakness in the legs
- ▸ Poor balance and gait (walking coordination)
- ▸ Reduced reaction time
- ▸ Poor or impaired vision
- ▸ Poor or impaired hearing
- ▸ Drop in blood pressure with a quick change in posture (e.g., standing from a sitting position)
- ▸ Medical conditions that affect balance or strength, multiple medication use, medications that affect water balance in the body
- ▸ Risky environment: inadequate lighting, uneven flooring, unsecured carpets and rugs, obstacles, narrow walking paths
- ▸ Personal habits: improper or inappropriate footwear, outdated vision prescriptions, refusal to use assistive devices

Home Environment

Most falls (over 60 percent) occur in the home. Most falls occur on a single level of the house, usually when someone is moving about. Unsafe home environments are created by the presence of obstacles, a lack of handrails, narrow pathways, uneven or slippery flooring, and poor lighting.

- Obstacles in the home increase the risk of tripping and stumbling. Common obstacles include furniture in the middle of open living spaces, clutter on floor space, open doors, electric or phone cords, small throw rugs with loose edges, and small children or pets.
- Lack of assistive devices such as handrails on staircases and grab bars in bathrooms near toilets and in showers can reduce steadiness and make a fall more likely.
- Narrow pathways are more difficult to move in comfortably and can increase the risk of catching a foot or toe along a wall or doorway.
- Uneven or slippery flooring can make it easier to trip, stumble, or slip and harder to catch oneself. Unsafe floor surfaces include wet kitchen or bathroom floors, slick or warped wood floors, bathtubs, deep shag carpets, and abrupt transition zones (e.g., interface between a kitchen linoleum floor and a living room carpet).
- Poor lighting can increase the risk of running into an obstacle and falling. A lack of lighting, including dim lighting from sources such as night-lights, bedside lamps, or stairway lights, and a lack of accessible light switches makes it more likely that hazards will go unseen.

Personal Habits

Risky personal habits such as wearing improper footwear, refusing to use assistive devices, and excessive alcohol consumption can contribute to instability inside and outside of the home. Shoes with high or narrow heels and those that do not fit properly make for unsure footing. Refusal to use assistive devices such as canes and walkers prescribed to improve stability removes an effective fall-prevention strategy. (In fact, it was my grandfather's failure to use his walker during a midnight trip to the unlighted kitchen for a drink of water that caused him to fall and break a hip.) Excessive alcohol consumption can impair one's balance and ability to avoid obstacles.

Medical Conditions or Treatment

Physical changes resulting from a medical condition or its treatment may impair stability or cause weakness that leads to a fall. Ideally, you should consult with a medical professional and pharmacist who can evaluate which medical conditions or treatments may increase your risk of a fall and advise you on appropriate measures and medication adjustments to reduce risk. Medical conditions that may contribute to fall risk include musculoskeletal impairments such as arthritis; neurological conditions such as multiple sclerosis, Parkinson's disease, or stroke; cardiovascular disease that can affect blood pressure; bladder or urinary problems that lead to dehydration; and alterations in mental status such as depression or Alzheimer's disease. Research has shown that people who take more than four prescription medications or any psychoactive (mind-altering) medication are at higher risk of falling (Tinetti and Speechley 1989; Ray and Griffin 1990; Cumming 1998). Many prescription medications can alter balance either directly or by causing dehydration or interacting with other medications, including over-the-counter drugs. I cannot list all the potential balance-altering medications and potential interactions here, but your pharmacist is an expert who can advise you on this issue and recommend suitable solutions.

Aging

As we age, physical changes can cause declines in our ability to maintain balance and walk smoothly, in muscle strength, and in vision. Any one or a combination of these declines can increase the risk for falling. A recent research review highlighted muscle weakness in the legs as the most significant risk factor for falling among older adults (American Geriatrics Society et al. 2001). Close behind were impairments in balance and walking coordination. Changes in vision can impair the ability to see and navigate around objects in one's environment. The good news is that many of these declines can be mitigated with a targeted exercise program such as the one we present in chapter 6. Visual declines can also be lessened by updating visual prescriptions, seeing an ophthalmologist or optometrist, and improving lighting conditions in the home.

A decline in muscle strength, caused in part by loss of muscle mass, typically begins in our 30s and becomes more pronounced after age 60. Although these losses have been attributed to the aging process itself, reduced physical activity is also a likely contributor (Horber et al. 1996). As we age, we tend to do fewer activities that require muscle strength, such as lifting objects or climbing stairs, and this causes strength-producing muscle fibers to shrink. Loss of muscle strength affects our ability to balance and to recover from a fall once it has begun. To appreciate how much leg strength contributes to balance, try standing on one leg for 15 seconds and realize how much you must use your leg muscles to keep yourself stable. Stability also worsens with age, and although strength declines may partially explain this change, instability is likely caused by changes in many physical systems, including the visual system, the inner ear balance system, and the sensory systems.

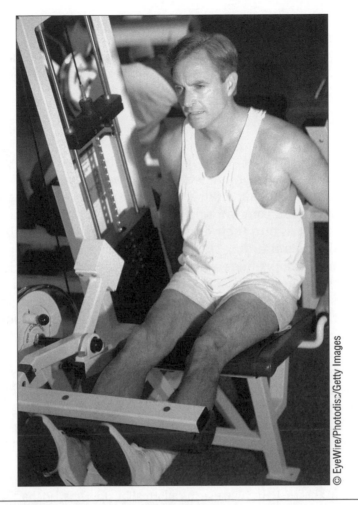

Muscle weakness in the legs is a prime factor in fall risk. Strength training can help improve balance and stability, thus helping to prevent falls.

Using Physical Activity to Prevent Falls

Physical inactivity accelerates age-related declines in muscle mass, strength, and balance. Thus, along with creation of a safe living environment and minimization of the side effects of medical conditions, physical activity aimed at improving strength and balance should lead to reduced risk of falling. In fact, most successful fall-prevention programs include at least some form of exercise as part of a broader prevention program. Exercise-only programs that target specific risk factors for falls, such as muscle weakness and poor balance, have also been successful in reducing falls (Sherrington et al. 2004). In survey studies, older adults who report being moderately physically active (accumulating 30 minutes or more of moderate-intensity activity most days of the week) have a lower risk of falls. Physical activity is an important part of a healthy lifestyle that includes lowered risk of injury from a fall. Chapter 6 includes an exercise program based on the latest scientific research that specifically tackles fall risk factors and best reduces your fall risk.

Summary

Falls are a significant risk factor for fracture. Some advocates argue that fall risk should be given equal weight with bone density when it comes to evaluating fracture risk. A fall is rarely the result of a single risk factor. More often several factors working together, and ultimately the interaction between individuals and their environment, determine whether they will sustain a fall. Understanding the modifiable risk factors for falls will help you construct a comprehensive strategy to best lower your risk of falling. Physical factors such as muscle weakness and poor gait and balance are often at least partially responsible for a fall. Even moderate amounts of physical activity can lower your fall risk and should be considered in any plan to reduce your risk of falls.

▷ *Personal Fall Risk Inventory*

Following is a list of known risk factors for falling. Most falls are the result of multiple factors. Since most people have more than one risk factor, being able to identify those that are most pertinent to you will give you the best information for creating a targeted and effective set of fall-prevention strategies.

Simply run down the list of risk factors and place a check mark or an *X* next to the statements that apply to you. Then use the information presented in the "Fall-Reduction Strategies" box on page 20 to learn about ways to reduce your fall risk. *You may also wish to consult with your physician on medically related risk factors.*

ENVIRONMENT

_____Furniture or clutter (plants, magazines) placed in the middle of a room

_____Phone or electric cords lying across traffic areas

_____Throw rugs that are not tacked down or otherwise secured

_____Pets that lie at your feet or follow you around the house when you move

_____Low lighting in traffic areas such as the bedroom, bathroom, hallways, and stairways; insufficient night-lights or light switches located too far away for easy access

_____Handrails not on both sides of the staircase

_____No grab bars installed in bathroom near toilet or in shower

_____Narrow walking paths due to cluttered spaces or poorly placed furniture

_____Slippery surfaces in or around the house, such as slick flooring, bathtubs, wood or worn carpeted staircases, icy walkways

_____Uneven floor surfaces such as deep shag carpet, warped or damaged tile or wood flooring, transition zones where floor surfaces change abruptly

PERSONAL HEALTH AND HABITS

_____History of cardiovascular disease, including hypertension

_____History of neurological disease such as multiple sclerosis, Parkinson's, or stroke

_____History of depression or other cognitive impairment such as dementia

_____History of muscle, bone, or joint disease such as arthritis, Grave's disease, or osteoporosis

_____Current bladder or urinary problems

_____Wearing unstable shoes such as those that have high heels or slick soles, are too small or too big, or do not support the heel

_____Refusal to use assistive devices such as canes, walkers, or safety bars and railings

_____Excessive alcohol consumption (more than three drinks daily)

PHYSICAL HEALTH

_____Inactivity. This equates to less than 30 minutes per day of moderate exercise most days of the week.

_____Noticeable muscle weakness in the legs. You may recognize this condition by a reduced ability to rise from a seated position, fatigue when climbing stairs or walking on an incline, or a feeling of unsteadiness while standing.

_____Poor balance. You may be able to recognize this condition on your own, in that you often need to grab onto something to steady yourself, or you can test this by timing how long you can stand on one foot. People who cannot stand on one foot for more than five seconds are more likely to fall. If you are at all unsteady, there is no need to try this test.

_____Poor walking coordination. You or someone who watches you may recognize this by a walking style that is slow, shuffling, or wobbly (side to side).

_____Poor vision. In particular, you may notice a reduced ability to see objects that are not immediately in front of you (i.e., peripheral vision) or to discriminate between different colors or surfaces.

Fall-Reduction Strategies

After evaluating your fall risk profile using the Inventory, consult the following list of strategies to address the risk factors present in you and your environment. *You are also urged to consult with your physician on medically related risk factors.*

ENVIRONMENT

▸ Declutter all rooms. Make clear paths for walking, and move obstacles such as furniture either out of the room or against a wall and away from traffic paths.

▸ Move all devices with cords that lie in traffic areas out of pathways or cover cords with floor coverings specially made for this purpose.

▸ Consider switching to wireless devices such as wireless phones and computer systems to eliminate cords.

▸ Tack down or remove throw rugs.

▸ Be aware of pets when you are moving about.

▸ Improve lighting in low-lit areas and those that are used during the night. Add night-lights (many are motion sensitive), light switches positioned for easy access, and tracking lights in hallways and on stairs or stairwells.

▸ Install handrails on both sides of the staircase.

▸ Install grab bars in the bathroom near the toilet and in the shower.

▸ Eliminate slippery surfaces in or around the house, such as slick flooring, bathtubs, wood or worn carpeted staircases, and icy walkways.

▸ Address uneven floor surfaces such as deep shag carpet, warped or damaged tile or wood flooring, and transition zones where floor surfaces change abruptly.

PERSONAL HEALTH AND HABITS

▸ Have a physical exam to check for diseases or conditions that may increase fall risk (see the Inventory for such conditions).

▸ Wear properly sized, stable shoes with low or no heels, traction on the soles, and heel support (athletic and walking shoes are good choices).

▸ Use assistive devices such as canes, walkers, and safety bars and railings.

▸ Limit alcohol consumption to fewer than three drinks daily.

PHYSICAL HEALTH

▸ Begin a physical activity program with the goal of achieving 30 minutes per day of moderate exercise most days of the week. It is okay to start with low levels of exercise and increase the duration and effort of activities over time.

▶ Incorporate the strength and balance exercises detailed in chapter 7 into your physical activity program at least two times per week. Balance exercises can be done every day and strengthening exercises up to four times per week.

▶ Have your vision fully evaluated and take corrective actions, including updating eyewear as needed.

ACTION PLAN:
FINDING WAYS TO PREVENT FALLS

☐ Know that falling is a strong risk factor for fracture, particularly for those with osteopenia or osteoporosis.

☐ Understand the risk factors for falling.

☐ Evaluate your risk of falling by completing the Personal Fall Risk Inventory.

☐ Adopt strategies for reducing fall risk (see "Fall-Reduction Strategies").

☐ Incorporate strength and balance exercises into your exercise routine.

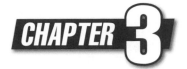
UNDERSTANDING THE RIGHT WAY TO APPROACH ACTIVITY

Now that you've taken the first step toward improving your bone health by learning more about osteoporosis, the next step is to become familiar with the basics of exercise training. Having a basic understanding of exercise training is central to being able to start your own exercise program or improve or update one that you've been using. Important concepts include the components of physical fitness, the principles of exercise training, the key elements of an exercise program, and safety precautions. After reading this chapter, you should have the building blocks necessary to construct any exercise program, whether you are currently inactive or are an exerciser looking to revise your program to address bone health. The information in this chapter will give you a preview of the framework for the sample exercise programs outlined in chapter 6. But keep in mind that these sample programs may not exactly fit your needs and cannot extend over long time periods. Thus, to build and maintain a regular program for many years to come, you will need the skills to tailor your program to your own likes, needs, and abilities. Next I'll describe the building blocks you need for managing your active lifestyle.

Components of Physical Fitness

When we say that someone is physically fit, what exactly do we mean? Do we mean they are strong? Fast? Flexible? Lean? Must a person have more than one or all of these attributes to be considered physically fit? The concept of physical fitness is rather broad but has been broken down into categories that describe distinct capabilities of the human body that decline with inactivity but can be honed with exercise. These categories are aerobic fitness, muscle fitness, flexibility, and body composition.

Aerobic Fitness

Aerobic fitness describes the ability of the heart and lungs to deliver oxygen and nutrient-rich blood to the muscles and for the muscles to use oxygen and nutrients to produce the energy for muscle contraction. The term *aerobic* refers to the way oxygen is used to help produce energy. When we move our body, our heart, lungs, and muscles are challenged to increase their rate of activity to keep up with the increased energy demands of exercising muscle. If we challenge our heart, lungs, and muscles on a routine basis through regular exercise, they adapt to become more efficient—or more "aerobically fit." Aerobically fit people can exercise at a higher level with less effort and can exercise longer, which has obvious benefits for athletes. But the adaptations that occur from regular aerobic exercise (defined later) also have significant health benefits for the average person and even the chronically ill. Regular aerobic exercise has been shown to decrease the risk of heart disease and related fatalities, prevent and manage diabetes and arthritis, improve bone health, decrease fall risk, improve blood lipids (e.g., increase good cholesterol), lower blood pressure in people with hypertension, and improve mood. For those who have become deconditioned due to prolonged periods of inactivity, bed rest, or illness, exercise can help restore the ability to perform tasks of daily living that may have become difficult.

Muscle Fitness

Muscle fitness refers to the ability of muscles to lift a lot of weight one time, called *muscle strength*, or many times, called *muscle endurance*. An example of someone who relies on muscle strength would be a moving man who needs to be strong enough to lift a refrigerator onto a dolly to move it into a house. A construction worker needs muscle endurance to drive nails into board after board with constant force. Muscle strength is obviously important for athletes such as power lifters or football linemen. But muscle strength is also important for everyday activities such as rising from a chair, getting out of bed, and moving furniture around, as well as for stopping ourselves from falling to the ground if we slip, trip, or stumble. Muscle endurance can be important for athletes such as downhill skiers, who have to contract their muscles for an entire downhill run, but it is also used in daily activities such as carrying groceries or grandchildren, painting a wall, gardening, or climbing the stairs. As with aerobic exercise, regular resistance training that challenges the muscular system helps us perform our daily and recreational activities and has additional health benefits, including maintenance of muscle mass, improved bone health, reduced fall risk, and lower blood pressure.

Flexibility

Flexibility is the ability of our muscles and joints to move through a range of motion. Good flexibility allows us to reach above or in front of us, to reach down and tie our shoes, to turn our head to look behind us while driving, and so forth. Of course, an athlete such as a gymnast is the quintessential example of a flexible person. We don't have to be able to bend over backward, though, to benefit from improved flexibility. Regular flexibility training (usually some form of stretching) improves our range of motion and allows us to perform our daily activities, to move safely in our environment, and to reduce our risk of an injury from sudden movement. Because of its steady pace and slow, controlled movements, flexibility exercise also makes us feel relaxed and less anxious.

Body Composition

Body composition describes the amount of fat and muscle mass in our body and is usually described as the percentage of our total mass that is fat, or our percent body fat. Body composition is measured using several different techniques that have varying levels of accuracy. If you have your percent body fat measured, be sure to ask the test technician how accurate and reliable the instrument being used is. When an athlete is described as "lean," that usually means she has a lot of muscle or not much fat. Someone who has a high percent body fat can have either a high amount of fat relative to muscle or a low amount of muscle relative to fat. The former example describes someone who may be at higher risk for chronic diseases linked to higher levels of body fat, including heart disease, stroke, diabetes, high blood pressure, and possibly some cancers. The latter example describes someone who may be at risk for conditions linked to low muscle mass, including poor physical function, poor bone health, or increased fall risk.

Typical ranges of percent body fat are 10 to15 percent for college-aged men and 20 to 25 percent for college-aged women (Lohman 1982). Research is less clear about what levels of body fat are associated with adverse health effects. Much of the relationship between fatness and health is based on a measurement called body mass index. Regular exercise training can alter body composition by reducing body fat or increasing muscle mass. Different types of exercise may be more effective at reducing body fat or increasing muscle mass. More on that later.

For most people, having their body fat measured is impossible due to lack of access to testing or because having this test done is too daunting an endeavor. However, one index of body fatness, referred to as the body mass index, or BMI, can be easily obtained from an individual's height and weight. BMI is correlated with percent body fat and can be used in the same way to indicate the presence of excess weight or obesity as a risk factor for certain chronic diseases. To determine your BMI, measure your height and weight as accurately as you can and use the following equation:

BMI = [weight in pounds ÷ (height in inches × height in inches)] × 703

For example, if a woman is 5 feet, 4 inches tall and weighs 140 pounds, her BMI would be 24.0, using the calculation

$$[140 \div (64 \times 64)] \times 703 = 24.0$$

Weight classifications associated with a given range of BMI are listed in table 3.1. A limitation of BMI is that it does not measure body fat directly, so in some individuals the relation between BMI and body fat is not as close. For example, at a given BMI, women may have a higher percent body fat than men and older people may have a higher percent body fat than younger people (Gallagher et al. 1996).

Table 3.1 Body Mass Index Ranges and Weight Classifications

BMI	Weight status
Below 18.5	Underweight
18.5 to 24.9	Normal
25.0 to 29.9	Overweight
30.0 and above	Obese

Courtesy of the Centers for Disease Control and Prevention, U.S. Department of Health and Human Services.

In contrast to the disease risks associated with being overweight, having low body weight and thus low BMI levels is a risk factor for osteoporosis and falls. We know that body weight is a strong determinant of bone density, such that low body weight is associated with lighter (and thus weaker) bones. BMI levels that correspond to the "underweight" category may indicate low muscle mass that would increase the risk of falls. In the osteoporosis literature, a body weight less than 127 pounds is listed as a risk factor for low bone mass (NOF 2004).

Principles of Exercise Training

A few guiding principles of exercise training should be kept in mind when creating an exercise program and when trying to determine whether your program is working. These principles will help you understand why one exercise is recommended over another, how the amount of exercise you do is determined, and what result to expect from your exercise program after you've been doing it regularly.

Specificity

The principle of specificity states that the type of exercise should be chosen to best meet the desired goal of the exercise program. For example, if your goal is to increase aerobic fitness, you should choose exercise that challenges the heart, lungs, and muscles over exercise that challenges your flexibility. If a swimmer wants to swim a faster 100-meter breaststroke, her training is focused on practicing the breaststroke as fast as she can. She may include additional types of training that supplement her main focus, but she certainly doesn't do the bulk of her training practicing the butterfly stroke for long distances. If you want to improve your bone health, you need to choose exercise that is known to challenge the skeleton so it will become stronger. The only way we know which type of exercise works best is through systematic research. In the next chapter, we will summarize what is known from exercise studies about the type of exercise that best challenges the skeleton.

Overload

The overload principle states that the target system of interest must be sufficiently challenged for it to adapt to exercise training. For example, if someone who can run a mile in five minutes wants to break that time, he doesn't train by continuing to run five-minute miles. Because he can run at this pace, his body has clearly already adapted well enough to do so. If he wants to become faster, he will have to practice running faster than his five-minute record for shorter distances. This training will challenge his body to adapt to running faster, and when he attempts to break his record, he will likely be successful.

It is unlikely that the goal of your exercise program is to break record running times, but you want to be confident that the effort you are investing in your program is worthwhile. It always pains me to see people working out at a gym at such a leisurely pace that they are really just going through the motions and not challenging their bodies to improve. My husband used to get so caught up in reading the newspaper while exercising on a stationary bike at our gym that he was pedaling like a turtle. He kept asking why he wasn't losing the weight he hoped to, so I told him to drop the newspaper and get moving! Making an exercise program challenging enough to ensure that you'll benefit from it is important and respects the time and effort spent exercising. The term *overload* may sound a bit daunting and could easily be replaced with the word *challenge*. Again, the exercise research has given us a good indication of how much exercise is necessary to improve bone health. The same research gives us an idea of how little exercise we can get away with and still reap the benefits, if time is an issue.

Progression

The principle of progression states that an exercise program must continue to be challenging for you to keep improving. When you exercise regularly and challenge your body, it responds by becoming more efficient and stronger. Eventually, your body becomes very adept at meeting the demands of your exercise program—it has adapted. This is not unlike what happens when you go on a diet. When you cut back on calories, your body adapts by losing weight. Eventually, your body becomes used to operating at the lower calorie intake and it gets harder to take off weight. This is often referred to as a "plateau." If you want to lose more weight, you either have to cut back a few more calories or exercise a little more. This same phenomenon happens when you exercise train. If you want to see even greater improvements after your initial gains, your program has to *progress* by increasing the overload, or challenge.

An exercise program can progress in several ways so that it is continually challenging, and we'll discuss those later in this chapter. We have also built progression into the exercise programs outlined in chapter 6. Be aware that you may reach a point in your exercise regimen where you are pleased with the benefit you've received and simply want to maintain what you've gained (see figure 3.1). In this case, your program can remain fairly constant, and you may simply wish to vary things from time to time just to keep exercise interesting and fun.

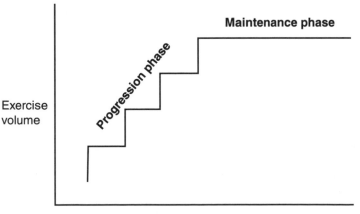

Figure 3.1 In the progression phase, exercise volume (the combination of frequency, intensity, and time) increases gradually over time to provide a constant challenge for the body to improve. At some point in training, the goals are reached, and the new goal of training is to maintain improvements by keeping exercise volume steady.

Reversibility

The reversibility principle could be easily renamed the "use it or lose it" principle. Simply stated, if you stop exercising, you will lose the benefits you gained from your exercise training. This principle may not necessarily hold true for young children who exercise, but unfortunately it does for adults. Even more distressing, though, is that the loss of benefits usually occurs twice as quickly as it took to gain them in the first place (Winters and Snow 2000). In our studies, we found that it took women one year to increase their hip bone density by 3 percent but only six months without exercise to lose most of that gain. The reversibility principle underscores the importance of finding an exercise program that you enjoy and that meets your specific needs, including the time and financial cost. We will consider these factors when talking about specific exercise programs in chapter 6.

Essential Measurements for Your Program

Every exercise program should include four essential components to ensure that it follows the principles of specificity, overload, and progression. These components are cleverly described by the acronym FITT, which stands for frequency, intensity, time, and type. I'll briefly describe each component and then give you a simple example of what a basic "exercise prescription" would look like. It's not as complex as you might think. Soon you will be able to develop your own prescription for improving your bone health.

Frequency

Frequency refers to the number of exercise sessions you perform over some time period. Frequency is typically expressed as *days per week* of exercise or, if you exercise more than once a day, as exercise *sessions per week*. Either convention is fine, but we will use days per week in our sample programs. Frequency is one of the components of a training program that can be manipulated to produce overload. Typically, for an adaptation to occur, we need to exercise somewhat regularly and at least two days per week, but the minimum and optimum frequency will depend on your starting level and your goals. Someone who has never strength trained before may start out with only one day per week of exercise, just to become familiar with such a program. Then, after she is more comfortable, she can progress to the recommended minimum of two days per week. Over time, she may really enjoy strength training and want to get stronger, so she can progress to three days per week, and so on. We also need to be careful not to overexercise, so some types of training are best performed every other day. We'll discuss those options in chapter 6 as well.

Intensity

Intensity refers to how much effort you put forth during exercise or how hard you exercise. Intensity is another component of training that can be manipulated to produce overload. Beginning exercisers should start off at a low intensity to ensure their safety and enjoyment of the initial program. After becoming more familiar with exercise, they can gradually increase the intensity to make the program more challenging and to see more benefit. In chapter 4, we'll discuss the recommended optimal range of exercise intensity to produce bone benefits.

Intensity is generally described as some fraction of your maximum capability, assuming this can be measured. Using this convention, exercise intensity can be adjusted for every individual. A one-fits-all intensity does not take into account that people differ greatly in their initial ability to perform exercise. For example, if I were to prescribe a walking program for a group of older women, they would likely start off with slightly different capabilities. Some may be slightly older than others, some slightly more fit, and some may have conditions that limit their ability to exercise. If I prescribe the exercise program for the group such that everyone has to walk at a pace of three miles per hour, some women won't be able to keep up and will be exercising near their limit and others will find the pace too slow and probably not challenging enough. It would be more beneficial to prescribe the exercise program according to their starting capabilities, for example, 50 percent of their top capacity. For women with a low starting capability, this may mean walking at two miles per hour, and for those with higher capability, it may mean walking at three miles per hour. Prescribing intensity in this relative way ensures that everyone is exercising at the level of effort that is right for them and is safe, yet challenging. Next, we'll discuss how to determine the intensity that is right for you.

Intensity is expressed in many ways and usually differs according to exercise type. For aerobic exercise, intensity can be expressed in the following ways: (1) percent of your maximal heart rate that is either determined from a test or estimated from your age, (2) percent of the maximum amount of oxygen you use during heavy exercise as determined by a test, or (3) self-rating of your effort, which we will discuss in chapter 6. For resistance exercise, intensity is referred to as a percentage of the highest weight you can lift as determined from a test called a one-repetition maximum (1 RM), where the weight you can lift once and once only is measured. Alternatively, the intensity of training can simply be set by the amount of weight you can lift a given number of times, such as a 6-repetition maximum weight or 10-repetition maximum weight, or a percentage thereof. Intensity of resistance exercise can also be rated subjectively, as for aerobic exercise. Resistance exercise for the lower body can also simply use body weight as a measure of effort. Raising your body out of a chair, for example, requires that your leg muscles work *against* the weight of your body to lift you up and out. To make this exercise more challenging, you could wear a *weighted vest* (described in chapter 7) that in effect increases the weight of your body and provides more resistance during a chair stand. Using this convention, intensity may be expressed as a *percent of your body weight* added to the vest. We used this method of overload in our exercise studies, and women gradually increased their intensity of resistance exercise from 1 percent of their body weight added to the vest on up to 15 percent of their body weight at the end of the program. Thus, someone who weighs 150 pounds would have gone from 1.5 pounds of added weight to 22 pounds of added weight over one year of exercise.

Other types of exercise we'll discuss are flexibility and impact exercise. For flexibility exercise, we express intensity as a self-rating of effort during a stretch—usually to the point of mild discomfort but not pain. For impact exercise, we usually use our body weight as resistance, but wearing a weighted vest during impact exercise, for example, could be used to increase intensity.

Any of these methods of determining and evaluating the intensity of your exercise program is acceptable, and we will discuss the advantages and disadvantages of each. Regardless of the method, you need to have some index of how hard you are working to ensure that you are working hard enough for the exercise to be of benefit but not so hard that you risk injury.

Time

Time refers to how much exercise you do in one session. Time is also termed the *duration* of exercise. As with the other components, time can be varied to produce the right amount of challenge for you. A beginning exerciser might start an aerobic exercise program by doing 10 minutes of aerobic exercise, two or three days per week. After a few weeks, she could gradually increase the time by 5 minutes a day so that she's worked up to 15 minutes per session. After another month, she could move up to 20-minute sessions, and so forth. The common convention for expressing time is the length of the exercise session in minutes, but time could also be expressed as a distance if you are someone who wants to walk or jog one to two miles per day. Obviously, time and distance cannot be used to measure the amount of resistance, flexibility, or impact exercise, so we use another convention. Because these types of exercise are done with multiple repetitions of a single exercise, we express time as the number of repetitions and the sets of repetitions. For example, an exercise prescription for impact exercise might begin with performing a total of 20 jumps per session, where 5 jumps in a row are completed (five repetitions) four separate times (four sets) with a short rest period between sets.

Type

Type refers to the kind of exercise you will do. Conventionally, type is called the *mode* of exercise. The type of exercise is chosen to fit the goal of the exercise program, following the *principle of specificity*. General types of exercise include aerobic, resistance, flexibility, balance, and impact exercise.

Aerobic exercise is any activity that uses the large muscle groups (entire upper body or entire lower body or both) and stimulates the heart and lungs (causes an increase in heart rate and breathing rate) over a continuous time period (usually a minimum of 10 minutes). Some common examples of aerobic exercise are walking, jogging, swimming, cycling, and dancing. Other forms include cross-country skiing, hiking, rowing, and marching in place.

Resistance exercise is any activity in which the muscles have to work against some type of force. Resistance exercise can also be called strength exercise or weight lifting, since weights are often used to provide the force, or *resistance*, against which the muscles must work. Resistance exercise typically uses some type of equipment to create resistance, such as weight machines, free weights (barbells and dumbbells), elastic tubing or bands, or medicine balls. As discussed earlier, our own body weight can be used to apply resistance to movement as well.

When we think about types of exercises to do, flexibility, balance, and impact exercise do not always pop to mind, but they can provide important health benefits. Flexibility exercise is that in which a part of the body is moved throughout its range of motion. Stretching is the most common form of flexibility exercise, but other types of exercise such as yoga or tai chi include some movements that challenge our flexibility. Balance exercise is that which challenges your ability to maintain an upright posture while standing or when in motion. Specific balance exercises can be performed or incorporated into other types of exercise, as is often done in yoga and tai chi. Impact exercise is a somewhat new classification of exercise based on findings that impact forces provide a challenge to the skeleton (discussed in more detail in chapter 4). Impact exercise is exercise that provides a quick burst of force when your feet or another body part make contact with the ground. Specific impact exercise includes movements such as jumping, hopping, or skipping that could also be incorporated into other activities (e.g., aerobic dance, stepping routines, basketball, volleyball, or gymnastics).

Warm-Up and Cool-Down

Although not part of the FITT acronym, a proper warm-up and cool-down are key components of any daily exercise session. A warm-up is an activity performed just prior to the main part of your exercise program that helps prepare your body for exercise. Warming up before exercise is similar to warming up your car in cold weather before you hit the road. Driving off too quickly can put more wear and tear on your engine, just as starting to exercise without warming up could put you at risk for injury. A proper warm-up before formal exercise helps increase the delivery of oxygen and nutrients to your muscles and warms them up so that they are more pliable. A typical warm-up includes some type of general activity that increases your heart rate about 10 to 20 beats above your resting pulse. This could mean simply exercising at a slightly lower intensity for the first 5 to 10 minutes of your session and then increasing the intensity during your main activity. For example, an aerobic dance class often begins with marching in place and circling the arms before starting more vigorous movements. For resistance exercise, the first set could be done with lighter weight and for more repetitions, and then the weight and repetitions increased on the next set or two. In my resistance exercise classes, we spend the first five minutes walking briskly around the room before we start lifting weights. Always remember to ease into exercise to avoid getting hurt.

A cool-down is an equally important part of any daily exercise session. The goal is just opposite that of the warm-up—to transition the body from exercise back to rest. When we are exercising, our bodies are working at a much higher level than usual, and stopping abruptly could be dangerous, particularly as we get older. During dynamic activity (where the arms and legs are continually moving), blood is moving very quickly throughout the body but, due to gravity, has a tendency to settle in the lower body if movement suddenly stops. This pooling of blood in the legs makes it more difficult for the blood to get back up to the brain to keep you alert. A lack of blood flow to the brain causes dizziness and confusion that could make you unstable and likely to fall. This phenomenon is more likely to occur in older people or those who are inactive. To prevent blood from pooling when you stop a dynamic activity, you need to lower your pace of exercise gradually until your heart rate starts to return to normal. Going back to the aerobic dance class example, the pace of the movements often slows to stepping in place before completely stopping exercise. A jogger might walk a lap on the track after jogging for 12 laps. For those who want to work on flexibility, the cool-down phase is also the best time to do some stretching exercise because the muscles are warmed from activity and tend to stretch farther. Stretching exercise can also be relaxing and provide a nice transition from an exercise session back to a hectic day. Stretching can be an effective cool-down after resistance exercise, where the need to slow down from dynamic movement does not apply but the need to stretch after working your muscles does.

Sample Aerobic Exercise Prescription Using FITT

▸ Begin with one lap of slow walking (warm-up)

▸ Alternate walking one lap with jogging one lap on high school track (type)

▸ 25 to 30 minutes a day (time)

▸ Three days per week (frequency)

▸ Use a pace that makes you feel slightly winded but able to talk (intensity)

▸ End with one lap of slow walking followed by upper and lower body stretches (cool-down)

Summary

Physical fitness is a body state that is important for athletic performance *and* for optimal health. Several aspects of physical fitness have important health implications. A comprehensive program that strives toward physical fitness should incorporate types of exercise that target all areas of fitness. An effective exercise program embraces the basic principles of exercise training. These principles apply even to a simple walking program undertaken with the aim of producing particular results in return for a given amount of effort. These principles help ensure that the work you are doing is paying off and helping you achieve your goals. Certain components of exercise training should be considered when embarking on any exercise program. The FITT principle is an easy way to remember that you should plan out the frequency, intensity, time (duration), and type of exercise training, as well as warm-up and cool-down periods. The timeline for exercise training will depend on your initial fitness level and health goals.

ACTION PLAN:
UNDERSTANDING THE RIGHT WAY TO APPROACH ACTIVITY

☐ Identify the components of physical fitness.

☐ Learn the principles of training.

☐ Become familiar with the methods for gauging exercise intensity.

☐ Know the essential components (FITT) of any training program, including the warm-up and cool-down.

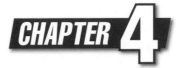

CHAPTER 4

LAYING A FOUNDATION FOR BONE HEALTH THROUGH EXERCISE

In the past two decades, much scientific research has been devoted to studying how exercise can reduce the risk of fracture by improving bone health and preventing falls. Only through well-controlled and well-designed studies can we be sure that a particular type and amount of exercise does what we expect it to. These studies can tell us if one type of exercise is more effective than another, how little exercise one can do and still reap benefits, and whether or not more exercise is better. Understanding all the research that has been published and deciphering the scientific jargon can be difficult. In this chapter, I'll review those studies in a way that will help you understand the scientific basis for the exercise programs described in chapter 6. I will summarize the research that has been done to date in an understandable way so that exercise makes sense!

Why Exercise Strengthens Bones

You have probably heard time and again that exercise must be "weight bearing" if it is to benefit your bones. How do we know that we must bear our weight during exercise? Why aren't swimming or bicycling, where our weight is supported by the water or by the bike, recommended as exercises for the skeleton? Some of the first evidence that weight bearing was important to the skeleton came from observations of bone loss in astronauts. When astronauts went into space, they lost bone and they lost it fast—at a rate of about 1 percent every month! This is 12 to 24 times faster than the rate at which we lose bone due to aging. Clearly, when we are upright, the invisible force of gravity puts a lot of stress on our bones every day. When we remove those stresses through immobilization (as when a leg is in a cast), long periods of bed rest (due to prolonged illness), or being inactive, bone mass can be lost. Similarly, non-weight-bearing exercises such as swimming or cycling may not be best for strengthening bones because the body weight is supported by the water or the bike instead of gravity.

When athletes who participate in weight-bearing sports are compared with athletes in sports that are non-weight bearing, the latter tend to have bone mass values similar to their peers who aren't athletes. On the other hand, athletes whose sports are weight bearing, and in particular athletes who place extra force on their bones through a lot of jumping or heavy weight lifting, tend to have the strongest skeletons. For example, swimmers and cyclists have bone mass values nearly equal to normally active people, whereas gymnasts, volleyball players, basketball players, and body builders have bone mass values that are up to 30 percent higher than inactive people (Fehling et al. 1995)! It appears that the skeleton gets stronger when it bears weight during exercise and when some amount of challenge (stress) is presented. Athlete studies indicated that various types of activities might be more or less effective at improving bone health. The one drawback to these studies, though, is that, by design, we cannot say for certain that exercise caused the differences in bone density. Because we cannot say for sure that athletes with lighter skeletons make better swimmers and cyclists and those with denser bones make better gymnasts and volleyball players, we need to look at studies where inactive people began different exercise programs and see which programs improved their bone health. Athlete studies provided the basis for the design and testing of exercise interventions aimed at improving bone health. These interventions can better answer the questions of what type and how much exercise strengthens bones. Recently, a summary report on exercise recommendations was prepared by a panel of experts from the American College of Sports Medicine to form a Position Stand on Physical Activity and Bone Health (Kohrt et al. 2004). Furthermore, the Surgeon General recently issued a national report on bone health, including important lifestyle modifications (such as exercise) for improving bone health, which can be accessed from the Web site: www.surgeongeneral.gov/library/bonehealth. The information in these important papers and careful review of the research form the basis for the exercise recommendations and sample programs covered in this chapter.

Determining the Most Effective Exercise for Bone

Exercise intervention studies help answer questions about the type and amount of exercise that is necessary to improve bone health. Bone health can be improved by increasing bone mass or by preventing or slowing the bone loss that typically occurs as people age. Increasing or preserving bone mass can translate to significant reductions in fracture risk, particularly when these effects are compared to the typical loss of bone mass that occurs with age. Various exercise studies have been conducted in women who had either normal, impaired, or poor bone health at the beginning of the exercise program. All three groups are important to study because they not only help us determine the right exercise program, but they also help us gauge whether exercise is possible and safe in those who already have osteoporosis or who have had a fracture. Compared to the research on women with normal bone mass, fewer studies of osteoporotic women have been done, but we can use this limited information along with standard safety precautions to set proper exercise limits and guidelines.

Keep in mind that I am only discussing the research studies that specifically tested exercise effects on bone. Although an exercise program may not be found to improve bone health, it probably has other important benefits that could be helpful to you. You could include several types of exercise in a lifelong exercise program that addresses your priority health areas. For example, if you have osteoporosis but also know that you are at risk for heart disease and are slightly overweight, you may choose to exercise specifically for your bones and muscles a couple of days a week and specifically for your heart and weight a few days a week. You would be wise to consider a well-rounded exercise regimen because varying exercise types can also prevent boredom and injury. In later chapters, we will outline what types of exercise and how much you need to do to improve bone health and reduce fracture risk so that you can include them in your lifestyle approach to optimizing your total health!

Traditional types of exercise have been studied for their bone health benefits, including weight-bearing aerobic exercise (e.g., walking, jogging, stair stepping, aerobic dance), resistance (strengthening) exercise, and impact exercise (e.g., jumping). These studies show that *most* types of exercise can benefit your bones but some types are better than others and that some types must be done at a certain level of effort to be effective.

Aerobic Exercise and Bone Health

Aerobic exercise has been studied in women with normal and poor bone health and can improve *both hip and spine bone mass* or prevent and slow bone loss. However, aerobic exercise must be performed with moderate effort to be effective. The types of aerobic exercise that have a positive effect on bone include very fast walking, jogging, stair climbing or stepping, and aerobic dance (Wolff et al. 1999). Positive effects range from slowing of bone loss to gains in bone mass of up to 3 percent. The average benefit across studies is a 1 percent gain in bone mass. Though seemingly small, a 1 percent increase maintained over time may translate into a significant

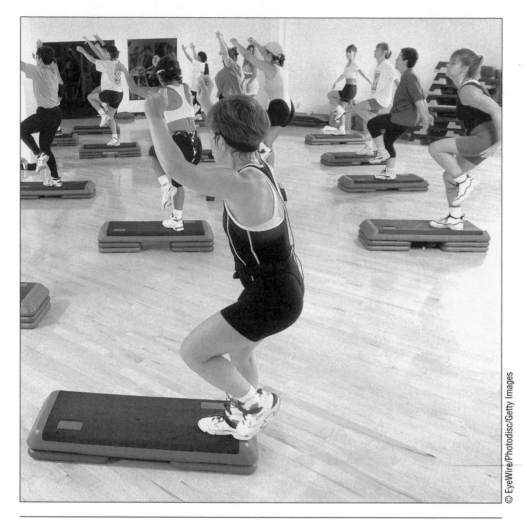

© EyeWire/Photodisc/Getty Images

Aerobic exercise that challenges the skeleton by putting stress on the bones is the most effective way to increase bone mass and slow bone loss.

reduction in fracture risk. This estimate is particularly true when a regular exercise program is initiated early and sustained for a lifetime.

The types of aerobic exercise that do not affect bone mass include slow or moderate-paced walking (less than three miles per hour) and aqua (water) aerobics. Other types of exercise that have not been studied include cross-country skiing, elliptical training, and hiking, so we cannot say for sure whether or not these exercises affect bone mass. Since walking is a weight-bearing exercise, you may be surprised to know that lower levels of walking may not benefit bone; I'll explain this more clearly in the sidebar on page 39.

Aerobic exercise has many other known benefits, including a reduction in heart disease and diabetes risk, improved functional ability (causing tasks to require less effort), weight maintenance or loss, lowered blood pressure, better blood lipids and blood sugar profiles, and improved mood and sense of well-being. Many people choose aerobic exercise because it is convenient, often requires little equipment or instruction, and can be done with a partner or in a group. Aerobic exercise may not provide the optimal level of benefit for muscle building or balance improvement, so if these are weak areas for you, consider adding some resistance and balance exercises to your aerobic program once or twice a week.

Is Walking Enough?

Walking is often advocated as a weight-bearing exercise that is good for bones. Large survey studies do show that women who walk fracture less often compared to women who are inactive. However, because of the way these studies are designed, they cannot establish that walking *causes* a reduction in fractures, nor can they tell whether walking may lower fractures because of its effect on bone or through other means. These studies can only show associations between walking and fractures, so it is possible that walkers engage in other healthy behaviors such as better calcium intake or decreased smoking that could lower their fracture risk. Perhaps walkers fall less, or perhaps habitual walking over many years provides a bone benefit that cannot be measured in research studies of short duration (one year or less). Just a few walking studies have shown a positive effect of walking on bone mass. In these studies, women walked at a very fast pace, similar to the speeds achieved by race walkers. These speeds are much faster than the average walking pace reported by most women. Race walkers can walk five to six miles in an hour, much faster than the two to three miles per hour for most women. Thus, if you plan to remain a walker and need to improve the health of your bones, you will probably need to ramp up the intensity of your walking program.

The fact that moderate-paced walking doesn't directly improve bone health comes as a surprise to most women I speak to, and as a disappointment as well, because they love to walk and don't want to give it up. Now, I would *never* recommend that anyone give up walking! If walking is an exercise you enjoy, keep doing it, because walking has many health benefits for you. However, the research suggests that exercise must be a little more rigorous than moderate-paced walking for it to improve bone health. This is likely because the skeleton does not view walking as a new challenge. Since most of us walk during our day just to get around, our skeleton has adapted to that activity. Bone is actually smart in this sense, because we surely don't want to break a bone just from walking around! So simply adding an extra 30 minutes of leisurely walking per day to our daily routine may not not challenge the skeleton enough to increase bone mass. There is a workable solution that will keep you walking and help reduce your fracture risk. Simply adding some specialized exercises to a regular walking routine may be all you need to get the heart-healthy benefits of walking and the bone benefits of specific exercise. I present an example of such a routine in chapter 6. Alternatively, you could plan to increase the intensity of your walking program to include bursts of very fast walking or walking briskly up hills. A more rigorous walking program would not only help your bones, but it would burn some extra calories and keep your heart healthy.

Resistance Exercise and Bone Health

Resistance training, also called strength training, can have a positive effect on bone because the strong muscle contractions required to lift, push, or pull a heavy weight place stress on the bone. Muscles are attached to bones by tendons, a type of connective tissue, so the force generated by a contracting muscle is in turn felt by the attached bone. When bone feels a force upon it time and time again (as happens in regular exercise training), it responds by increasing bone mass so as to become stronger and better tolerate the strong muscle contractions. Exercise studies have used several different means of applying resistance to the skeleton, including resistance machines, free weights such as dumbbells and barbells, weighted vests for the lower body, and elastic tubing or bands. Studies also used varying amounts and intensities of exercise. Generally, resistance exercise using any means of applying resistance of sufficient intensity successfully maintains or slightly improves hip and spine bone mass in most women (Wolff et al. 1999). In women with osteoporosis, moderate resistance exercise has been directed at fall prevention and has been shown to prevent falls.

By strengthening muscles that are important for fall prevention, resistance training also strengthens the muscles that are important for good physical function in performing tasks that require some strength (e.g., lifting groceries or grandchildren, rising from a chair, climbing stairs). Strong leg muscles can also contribute to better balance and locomotion that reduce the risk of falls. When someone starts to fall, having strong muscles makes it more likely they can stop their fall by quickly putting out a leg to counteract the downward movement. There is also some evidence that resistance exercise can help lower blood pressure, improve blood lipids (cholesterol and triglycerides), and aid in weight reduction.

Resistance exercise often conjures up images of big, bulky muscles and overcrowded gymnasiums. These stereotyped images can turn people off to the notion of lifting weights. However, resistance training can be done anywhere with minimal equipment (for some exercises, no equipment is required) and can even be fun. When I was a graduate student, I recruited and trained 40 middle-aged women to do resistance and impact exercise three times a week for a year. Only a few of the women had ever lifted weights before and most were intimidated and skeptical of the program, but we plodded awkwardly through the first weeks with a few grunts and groans, and after a month the women were hooked! They started feeling better and noticing the effects that having strong muscles had in their daily lives. One woman remarked that she could downhill ski better than she had in 20 years after doing our program regularly. Another found it easier to care for her husband, who had recently developed multiple sclerosis. And we did all of these exercises in a windowless, open room with very little equipment. I also led similar exercise classes for other studies in older and elderly women. They, too, were skeptical but after a month or two started noticing the difference. Women could garden with more ease and less stiffness and were able to hike the local mountains. Our elderly participants could take the stairs and get out of chairs without using their arms—tasks they swore they could never do. Most impressive of all is that many of these women have continued doing our exercise program, some for more than eight years now! They do the programs at home or in local fitness classes, but they swear they will never stop because they know the resistance exercise makes them feel better, benefits their bones, and lowers their risk of falling.

Resistance exercise is now recommended by the American College of Sports Medicine for all individuals, especially older adults who may have had some bone and muscle loss due to age. Following proper guidelines, resistance exercise has been safely performed even in 90-year-olds! Resistance exercise may be a new endeavor for you, but it could make a real difference in your life, so give it a try!

Impact Exercise and Bone Health

Impact exercise, usually performed as jumps, may offer a quick and simple way to improve bone mass at the hip. Hip fractures can be the most debilitating and costly of all fractures, so this is an important area to target. Jumping exercise works because it challenges the skeleton in a way that it does not typically experience. Most of us jumped around a lot when we were kids and occasionally do so as adults when we get excited, but typically we don't jump around much anymore. Jumping works because when we jump up and land on the ground, the force on landing is transferred up the skeleton. The skeleton perceives this force as a challenge and a stress to the system and responds by laying down more bone to better tolerate the stress of regular jumping. This adaptation is similar to what occurs in response to resistance exercise when strong muscle contractions challenge the bone.

Generally, studies have shown that women who perform jumping exercise, either alone or in addition to another exercise program such as walking or resistance training, maintain or improve their hip bone mass. We have studied the effects of jumping exercise plus resistance training in middle-aged and older adult women. Women who regularly engaged in resistance exercise plus 50 to 100 jumps, three times per week, increased or maintained hip bone mass; this included women with low bone density (Snow et al. 2000; Winters and Snow 2000). Unfortunately, jumping exercise alone does not appear to improve bone health of the spine because the forces generated on landing are so small by the time they reach the spine that there is insufficient challenge to these bones. Jumping exercise may be a singular program to improve bone health of the hip specifically or may be part of a total exercise program that targets both the hip and spine and produces other desired benefits such as cardiovascular health or muscle strengthening.

The thought of jumping exercise tends to conjure up images of little kids skipping rope or basketball players shooting jump shots. The latter is certainly a group that was found to have high bone mass, which in turn led to the theory that jumping exercise might improve bone health in the general population. Although for most of us, jumping exercise might seem silly or awkward, jump training has been used for years by athletes to help improve their jumping ability and power. Track athletes, volleyball players, basketball players, wrestlers, and gymnasts are just a few types of athletes who jump train to enhance their performance. Participating in jump training puts you in the company of these talented sportspeople. Many fitness classes are now adding jump training to "boot camp" or traditional aerobics classes to help improve bone and muscle. When results of our exercise studies were published in the local newspaper, I began seeing women jump during their workouts in the university gymnasium. If you are concerned about feeling self-conscious when jumping in public, don't be. Proudly tell those around you that you are exercising your bones and that there is scientific proof that it works! When my study participants had to travel, they were encouraged to exercise on the road. Many of these women jumped in hotel gyms, friends' homes, or outdoors. In fact, we even had a contest about the craziest place they had jumped. Women photographed themselves jumping on a beach in Hawaii, alongside Mickey Mouse at Disneyland, on top of Oregon's South Sister Mountain, and even in front of St. Peter's Cathedral in Rome—proof that you can jump anywhere, anytime!

Many of you may be concerned about the safety of jumping. This is a valid concern, and for some women, jumping may not be a viable exercise option. Safety concerns about jump exercise in women with osteoporosis are discussed in chapter 5. Women who have diagnosed orthopedic and joint limitations or who are significantly overweight should discuss jump exercise with their physician before starting a program and may wish to consider other types of exercise first. The injuries due to jumping exercise in our study and in others have been minimal. Some women complained of mild knee pain from exercise that was likely due to weak muscles around the knee joint. We could not tell if the pain was due to jumping or resistance exercise, but in these cases, the women cut back on their exercise temporarily and worked specifically on strengthening the muscles around the knees. After a few weeks, they were ready to jump and completed our program. Jumping exercise may not be for everyone, but some people love it and find it the quickest way to exercise their bones. Jumping only takes about 5 or 10 minutes to do, so it is easy to add to the end of a walk or jog and is an attractive exercise routine for people with limited time.

Determining the Proper Exercise Amount

The Healthy People 2010 public health initiative (along with similar efforts by the U.S. Surgeon General, the Centers for Disease Control, and the American College of Sports Medicine) recommends the following amounts of physical activity for adults (Pate et al. 1995):

- Adults should engage in *moderate-intensity* physical activities for at least 30 minutes on five or more days of the week.

or

- Adults should engage in *vigorous-intensity* physical activity three or more days per week for 20 or more minutes per occasion.

These guidelines fit within the scope of recommendations for improving your bone health and lowering your fracture risk. However, since they are rather general, I will add some detail to these recommendations based on research specific to bone health and summarized in the following paragraphs. Note that selection of exercise type should focus on weight-bearing activities.

Aerobic exercise studies suggest that exercise must be of moderate to high intensity to be effective. As discussed earlier, lower intensity exercise such as leisurely walking or easy cycling is unlikely to benefit bone. More vigorous aerobic exercise, such as very fast walking, jogging, running, or dancing (particularly when some form of stepping routine is included), that is weight bearing and is performed at a moderate to vigorous pace for 30 to 60 minutes three to five days per week should improve bone health.

Resistance exercise, too, must be slightly rigorous to affect bone. Low-intensity resistance training performed with light weight and for many repetitions generally is of no benefit. This type of exercise is often touted as "sculpting" or "toning" exercise and simply doesn't place enough force on the bones. Low-weight, high-repetition resistance exercise may be a good starting point for people who have never performed resistance exercise. (*Note:* Low weight is weight you could comfortably lift 15 to 20 times (15- to 20RM, or less than 60 percent of 1RM), and high repetition refers to three to five sets of 15 to 20 repetitions per set.) Beginning at this level, novices can become familiar with resistance training and start to build a base of strength from which they can progress to heavier weights (weight that cannot be lifted more than 8 to 12 times (8- to 12RM, or 70 to 85 percent of 1RM) lifted less often (two or three sets of 8 to 12 repetitions per set). We'll look at an example of this type of program in chapter 6. Most studies suggest that resistance exercise must be performed at least two times per week to be effective, although one study showed positive effects from one day a week of resistance exercise. For those who are new to this type of training, one day a week may be a good starting point for becoming familiar with the activity, ideally progressing to two or three days per week.

The appropriate overload for jump training has been studied far less. Most studies have women perform a variety of jumping routines, including simply jumping straight up and down. When the height of the jump

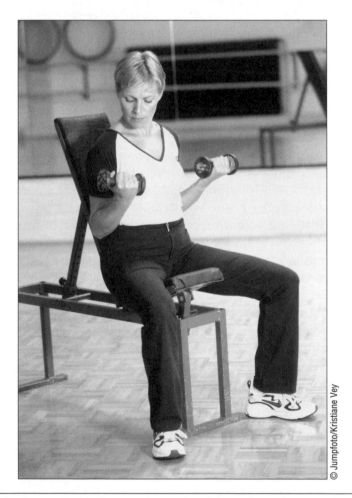

© Jumpfoto/Kristiane Vey

Strength training has optimal effects on bone when it is performed at a moderate intensity, two or three times per week.

(jumping onto and off of small steps) or the weight of the person jumping is increased (jumping while wearing a weighted vest), the jump produces more force. Our studies have shown that younger women who jump wearing a weighted vest and onto boxes increase their hip bone mass, but that older women who jump without a vest maintain their hip bone mass over time. Generally, 50 to 100 jumps in place done three to five days per week are recommended as a suitable routine based on the research. Jumps are usually done in multiple sets of 10.

You may also wonder how long you have to exercise before your bones start to benefit. Unlike other physiological systems such as the heart and muscles, which respond to exercise rather quickly, the skeleton takes its time. Because the process of bone building is slow, it takes at least six months before we can *measure* the effect of exercise. Rest assured that the bone-building process begins as soon as you start to exercise regularly, but it takes a while for us to be able to detect that change through bone mass (density) measurement. All exercise research studies are a minimum of six months in length and usually last for one year. This means that you must be patient yet persistent, and most of all, you need to find an exercise that you will stick to for a lifetime. We know that bone benefits from exercise are lost when someone stops training, so any exercise you do for your bones must be something you can commit to long term. Fortunately, you have many choices and are likely to find and begin such a program!

Exercise Specific to Fall Prevention

Because falls are a leading cause of fracture, along with weak bones, much exercise research has focused on fall prevention. If you have osteoporosis, fall prevention should be a major focus of your exercise program. Fortunately, the research has given us a pretty good idea of the type and quantity of exercise that will help prevent falls. Remember, though, that falls can have many causes, and exercise may be only one of several steps you take to lower your fall risk. Go back to the checklist in chapter 2 to determine what other important strategies you could adopt.

We know for certain that weak legs, poor balance, and difficult locomotion (also called *gait*) make one much more likely to fall than someone who is strong, stable, and moves about easily. Since muscle mass, strength, gait, and balance are all closely related to one another, most exercise intervention programs include strengthening exercise along with balance training. Resistance training programs are largely successful at increasing muscle mass and dramatically improving muscle strength in people who are weak to begin with and also bring about improvements in balance and gait. Resistance training, either with or without additional balance training, has been shown to reduce falls. Research studies of exercise that focused on balance only, without resistance exercise, generally did not prevent falls. Some nontraditional forms of exercise, more popular in Asian countries, have been shown to reduce falls and will be discussed in chapter 6. Together, all of these studies underscore the importance of strong muscles for fall prevention.

Summary

Scientific research has shown us that exercise can improve bone health by increasing bone mass or by slowing or preventing age-related bone loss. This same research has provided guidance for determining the type and quantity of exercise necessary to help maintain or boost bone health. Although leisurely levels of physical activity are good starting points for beginning an exercise program, more moderate to vigorous levels of activity are necessary to challenge the bones to become healthier. Exercise is also important for fall prevention, and certain types of exercise have been shown to be optimal in lowering fall risk.

ACTION PLAN:
LAYING A FOUNDATION FOR BONE HEALTH THROUGH EXERCISE

☐ Be confident that exercise can improve your bone health; scientific research has shown this to be the case.

☐ Have a general understanding of the types of exercise that improve bone health and their other important health benefits.

☐ Be aware that leisurely to moderately paced walking may not directly improve bone mass, but *very fast* walking, such as race walking, can improve bone mass of the spine.

☐ Know that exercise can also help lower your risk of falling.

☐ Understand that you must exercise at moderate intensity to benefit.

☐ Be assured that lower intensity exercise is a safe starting point for unfit or inactive individuals, who can then progress to a more moderate intensity program over time.

☐ Remember that exercise must be done consistently to reap the long-term benefits!

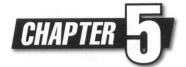

CHAPTER 5

EVALUATING YOUR BASELINE FITNESS

Evaluating your baseline fitness level is important for several reasons. Knowing where you're at allows you to identify your strong and weak areas and to develop a program that is not too difficult but challenging enough to be of benefit. It will also give you a reference point for determining whether you are achieving the desired results. For many of you, it may be enough to know that you have been inactive for some time, are probably unfit, and need to start exercising at a low level. Others of you may already be exercising regularly and are somewhat fit but want to further improve your fitness or work on your weak areas. Some of you may be unsure of your starting level for different fitness areas and want to establish a measurable baseline so that you can chart your progress.

In the next few pages, I'll discuss a couple of ways to establish your baseline level of aerobic fitness, muscle strength and endurance, flexibility, mobility (gait), and balance. Most of these tests are modifications of standardized laboratory tests that can be easily and safely performed at home, even by older people (Rikli and Jones 2001). These evaluations should be done with a partner, or at least with someone in the vicinity who can assist you if you accidentally fall or get injured, particularly if you are inactive or unsteady. If you are not confident that you can safely perform these basic evaluations, do not proceed unless you are supervised. Evaluation results can be recorded on the scorecard on page 57.

You do not have to do these evaluations before beginning an exercise program; they are only designed to add depth to your plan. Do not proceed with any test if you become dizzy, light-headed, or unsteady, or if you experience any sort of pain, including chest, arm, or jaw pain. If you experience any of these symptoms, consult your physician before continuing with an exercise program. Above all, use common sense.

Determining Your Baseline Aerobic Fitness

Simple running, walking, or stepping tests can be used to estimate your aerobic fitness and determine a baseline. Instructions for the 1.5-mile walk or run (ACSM 2000), the six-minute walk (Rikli and Jones 2001) test, and the two-minute step test (Rikli and Jones 2001) are given in the following sections. Percentile scores for these tests are listed in the appendix.

▷ *1.5-Mile Walk or Run*

The 1.5-mile walk or run is a timed test that measures how fast you can walk or run 1.5 miles. *This test is appropriate for someone who already regularly engages in moderate-intensity aerobic exercise such as brisk walking, jogging, or cross-country skiing.* You will need to do this test on a measurable course, such as a treadmill or high school quarter-mile track. Warm up at a pace slower than your estimated walking or running pace for about 5 to 10 minutes, then time how quickly you can walk or run 1.5 miles (six laps on the inside lane of a standard track). When you complete 1.5 miles, cool down by walking or jogging slowly for another 5 to 10 minutes and then stretch your hips and legs. You can predict an estimate of aerobic fitness, measured as the volume of oxygen (ml) consumed per kilogram (kg) of body weight per minute (min), called $\dot{V}O_2$max or maximal aerobic power, using the following formula:

$$\text{Predicted } \dot{V}O_2\text{max (ml/kg/min)} = 3.5 + 483/(\text{time in min})$$

This is your baseline aerobic fitness, and if you like, you can compare it to the norms listed in the percentile values for maximal aerobic power table in the appendix. You can repeat this test after you've been exercising regularly; you should be able to increase the distance you can walk or run as you become more fit.

▷ *Six-Minute Walk (6MW)*

The 6MW test has been used in many different populations, both healthy and ill, to evaluate aerobic fitness and is a good test for less fit or less active people. The test requires you to walk as far as possible in six minutes. You will need some way to measure the distance you walked, as you could by walking on a treadmill or nearby track, and you need to be able to measure time in minutes accurately. Once you've decided on a course, simply walk as far as you can in six minutes. You may want to walk slowly for a few minutes before starting to time yourself to make sure you are warmed up and ready to go. You will also need to pace yourself during the test since you need to keep walking for six minutes. When the six minutes are up, note how far you walked on a scorecard, and cool down with a slow walk and some stretching. If desired, you can compare your time to the norms listed in the appendix. This is your baseline aerobic fitness, and you can repeat this test after you've been exercising regularly; you should be able to increase the distance you can walk in six minutes as you become more fit. If you don't have access to a measurable course, you can perform a rough version of this test simply by tracking how far you walk on your usual course during a six-minute stretch where you push yourself. For example, if you can walk halfway around the block in six minutes when you start exercising, you can then see how many additional houses you can get past after walking regularly for a month. Although there are no norms for this method, it is a simple way to measure the progress of your fitness program.

▷ Two-Minute Step Test (2MST)

The 2MST is an alternative to the 6MW if you do not have a place to walk where you can accurately measure the distance traveled (Rikli and Jones 2001). For this test,

you count the number of steps you can take in place over a two-minute period. You will need to mark off the appropriate step height by placing masking tape on a wall, door, or chair. Place a piece of tape on the wall at a point midway between the top of your kneecap and the top of your hip bone. This is the height you should lift your knees to when you step in place during the test. Stand so that your right shoulder is perpendicular to the wall and give yourself a step or two of distance out from the wall (see figure 5.1). Using a watch with a second hand or a stopwatch, begin the test. For the next two minutes, step in place to the marked height and count one step each time your right leg reaches the tape mark (do not count one step for each knee). Write the number of steps you completed in two minutes on your scorecard. This is your baseline aerobic fitness, and if desired, you can compare it to the norms listed in the appendix. You can repeat this test after you've been exercising regularly; you should be able to increase the number of steps you complete as you become more fit.

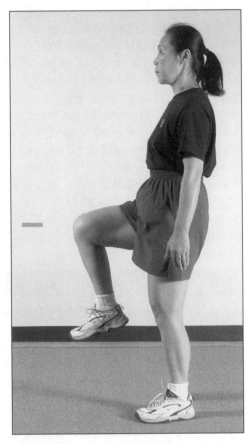

Figure 5.1   Proper position for the two-minute step test.

Determining Your Baseline Muscle Strength

Muscle strength can be evaluated in many ways. The test you choose will depend on how familiar you are with doing resistance exercise. In the following sections, I describe several ways to determine the strength of your upper and lower body.

▷ One-Repetition Maximum (1RM)

The 1RM is the gold-standard test for muscle strength (ACSM 2000). It is simply the highest amount of weight you can lift, push, or pull with your arms or legs one time only. It is often the index by which the amount of weight (intensity) is chosen for a strength training program, but intensity can be figured without using this test. *You should be reasonably fit and familiar with resistance exercise to do this test, and you should ALWAYS be tested under supervision.* What is helpful about this test is that it allows you to determine your strength for any muscle group. Typically, the bench press is used for testing overall upper body strength and the leg press for testing overall lower body strength. Obviously, this type of test must be done in a gym or similar community setting where equipment is available. Percentile rankings for these tests are included in the appendix.

You should first perform a warm-up with a weight you can easily lift 10 to 12 times and then increase the weight to one you can lift about 4 to 6 times. You can then estimate your test weight, which will take some guesswork. It will probably be at least two increments (an increment is typically 5 or 10 pounds) higher than the weight you just lifted. Select that weight and try to lift it. If you cannot, then decrease the weight and see if you can lift that. If you can lift the decreased amount of weight, this is your 1RM. If not, keep decreasing until you find your 1RM weight. If you can lift the first weight, take a few minutes' rest, then increase to the next increment and try again. Keep increasing the weight until you get to one that you cannot lift at all. At this point, the weight that you lifted just *before* this one is your baseline 1RM.

▷ Submaximal Tests of Muscle Strength: 6RM or 10RM

If you do not feel safe performing the 1RM, you can estimate your strength from a 6RM or a 10RM test. These "submaximal" tests of muscle fitness are indices of the strength and endurance of your muscles. The 6RM is the amount of weight you can lift 6 times and no more, and the 10RM is the amount of weight you can lift 10 times only. For the 6RM test, you warm up with a weight you can lift about 10 times and do 10 repetitions with that weight, and for the 10RM, you warm up with a weight you can lift 15 times and do 15 reps. Then bump up a couple of increments and try to find the weight for your 6RM or 10RM. A disadvantage of these tests is that, because you have to do some guesswork, you may end up lifting so many times that you get tired before you find your true 6RM or 10RM. Be sure to give yourself plenty of rest between attempts so that you can best estimate your true strength. Although it is difficult to estimate your 1RM from your 6RM or 10RM weight (Hoeger et al. 1987), doing so does provide a useful index of your muscle strength and endurance and can also help in determining your appropriate starting weight for a resistance training program, as discussed in chapter 6. If you use the 1RM method, you can compare this result to the percentile scores for 1RM listed in the strength tables in the appendix. You can repeat these tests after you've been exercising regularly; you should be able to increase your 1RM, 6RM, or 10RM weight as you become more fit.

▷ Sit-to-Stand and Arm Curl

The sit-to-stand and arm curl tests are measures of your lower and upper body muscle strength plus endurance, respectively. Since muscle endurance is related to muscle strength, these tests can give you an idea of your initial strength level. Norms for healthy community-dwelling adults 60 years of age and older are listed in the appendix (Rikli and Jones 2001).

SIT-TO STAND

The sit-to-stand test measures how many times you can rise from a seated position in 30 seconds. You need to have a straight-backed chair with sturdy legs (no wheels) and a stopwatch (it may be easiest to have someone else time you). Place the back of the chair against a wall for stability. Sit in the middle of the chair seat with your back straight and your feet flat on the floor, in line with your knees. Cross your arms across your chest and then start the stopwatch. Rise up from the chair to a full stand (legs and back straight) as quickly as possible and then return to a seated position as quickly as possible. Repeat for 30 seconds and write the number of times you stood up in that time period on your scorecard. You may want to practice standing and sitting once or twice before you test yourself to get the hang of it. To keep track of your stands, you may want to count out loud. You can repeat this test after you've been exercising regularly; you should be able to increase the number of stands you can complete as you become more fit.

ARM CURL

The arm curl test measures how many times you can lift a standard weight with your arms in 30 seconds. You need to have a straight-backed chair with sturdy legs (no wheels), a five-pound (women) or eight-pound (men) dumbbell, and a stopwatch (it may be easiest to have someone else time you). Place the back of the chair against a wall for stability. Sit slightly to one side of the chair seat (the side toward the arm you'll lift with) with your back straight and your feet flat on the floor, in line with your knees. Hold the weight down at your side, perpendicular to the floor, in a handshake grip (palm facing your seated leg). Curl the weight up, flexing at the elbow, until the weight is almost parallel to your shoulder, and then return your arm to the starting position. Your palm should turn up as you lift the weight and should turn back to the handshake position as you lower it (see figure 5.2). Your upper arm (the segment between your shoulder and elbow) must remain still throughout the test. Have someone watch you do an arm curl once or twice to make sure you are doing it correctly. Keep lifting and lowering the weight for 30 seconds and write the number of times you lifted the weight in that time period on your scorecard. To keep track of your curls, you may want to count out loud. You can repeat this test after you've been exercising regularly; you should be able to increase the number of times you can curl this weight as you become more fit.

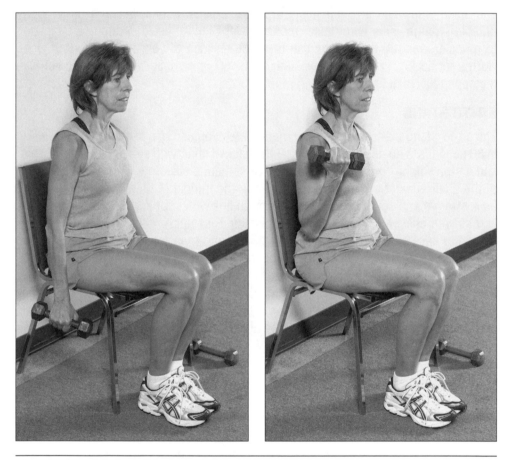

Figure 5.2 Proper technique for the arm curl test.

Determining Your Baseline Flexibility

Two simple tests—the sit-and-reach test and the back scratch test—can help you determine the flexibility of your lower and upper body, respectively (Rikli and Jones 2001). You can compare your baseline flexibility against age-established norms and can use your baseline to chart your progress.

▷ *Sit-and-Reach Test*

The sit-and-reach test measures the flexibility of your legs, primarily the muscles in the backs of your legs. Do not perform the stretches for this test rapidly or in a bouncy fashion, and stop the test if you feel any pain. You should feel a deep stretch but not pain! This version of the sit-and-reach test is performed in a seated position on a chair. You will need a yardstick or tape measure and preferably a partner to measure your performance. Sit in the middle of a stable chair that is positioned against a wall. Keep one foot flat on the floor and extend the other leg in front of you, with your heel on the floor, your foot flexed, and your knee slightly bent. Raise both arms overhead and place the palm of one hand on the back of your other hand. Take a deep breath, and as you exhale, reach your arms in front of you toward your feet (see figure 5.3). Slowly stretch as far as you can and measure the distance between the tip of your middle finger and your toes. Scoring for this test is as follows: If your fingertips are just touching the tip of your toes, your score is zero (0); if your fingertips are in front of your feet (closer to your body), it is counted as a minus score (e.g., –2.5 inches); if your fingertips go past your toes, it is counted as a plus score (e.g., +1.5 inches). Take two practice trials and then two test trials and record the better of the two test trials on your scorecard. You may want to test your flexibility on both legs, but only count your highest score for either leg as your flexibility score. Your highest score is your baseline lower body flexibility and can be compared against the norms listed in the appendix.

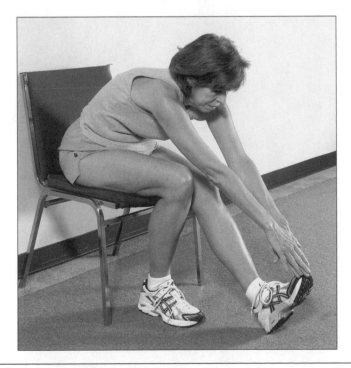

Figure 5.3   Proper position for the sit-and-reach test.

▷ *Back Scratch Test*

The back scratch test measures the flexibility of your upper body, mainly your arms and shoulders. You will measure how closely you can place your hands together behind your back. Do not perform the stretches for this test rapidly or in a bouncy fashion, and stop the test if you feel any pain. You should feel a deep stretch but not pain! For this test, you will need a second person to measure distance with a tape measure or yardstick. In a standing position, place your dominant hand over the same shoulder (e.g., right hand over right shoulder), palm down and fingers extended. Reach this hand as far as possible down the middle of your back, keeping your elbow pointed up. At the same time, place your other arm around the back of your waist with your palm up, then reach up the middle of your back as far as possible with this hand and try to touch or overlap the extended middle fingers of both hands (see figure 5.4). Scoring for either position is the same as for the sit-and-reach test. If your fingertips are just touching, your score is zero (0). If your fingertips do not touch, the distance between your fingertips is counted as a minus score (e.g., –2.5 inches). If your fingertips go past one another, the distance between your fingertips is counted as a plus score (e.g., +1.5 inches). Take two practice trials and then two test trials and record the better of the two test trials on your scorecard.

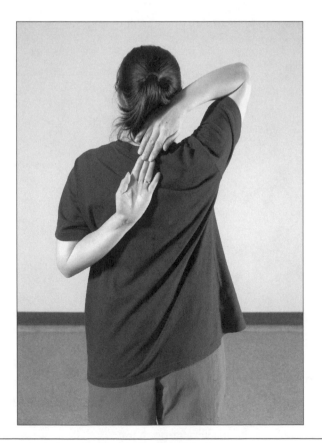

Figure 5.4 Proper technique for the back scratch test.

Determining Your Baseline Balance

The following balance tests measure how long you can keep yourself stable in either a one-legged position or a two-footed heel-to-toe stance. As there are no normative values for these balance tests, you will only be able to use them as a baseline for evaluating how your balance improves with exercise.

▷ *One-Legged Stand*

This test measures how well you can balance yourself while standing on one foot. People who fall generally cannot stand as long on one foot as people who do not fall. *Do not perform this test if you have a history of falling or are unsteady or lack confidence in your ability to perform the test. Instead, you should perform the tandem stance test or simply forgo testing.* You will need an open space that is free of obstacles and a stopwatch. You may want to position yourself close to a wall, so that you can steady yourself if you begin to lose your balance. Test yourself either with bare feet or wearing sturdy athletic shoes. When you retest yourself at a later time, you should use the same conditions as in the baseline test (shoes either on or off). Do not do this test wearing socks or dress shoes (if you're on a slippery surface, you may fall). Begin timing yourself once you have lifted one foot off the floor. Lift your foot off the floor by bringing your knee up slightly, just a little in front of you. You do not need to raise your knee very high or bring your raised foot far behind you. Time yourself until you put your foot down or 30 seconds have elapsed. If you start to shuffle or move your feet, the test is done. Write your time on your scorecard. This is your baseline balance. There are no norms for this test, but you can use it as a baseline for measuring your improvement. The time you can stand on one foot should increase as you become more fit.

▷ *Tandem Stance*

If you are unable to stand on one foot for any length of time, you can modify the one-legged stand test to a tandem stance test (Guralnik et al. 1994). This test is known to assess balance, and people who fall generally cannot maintain the tandem position as long as people who do not fall. Have someone supervise you while performing this test, and be sure to do the test in an obstacle-free, safe setting. For this test, you will time how long you can maintain a tandem, or heel-to-toe, position. Get into the tandem position and then time how long you can remain in the heel-toe stance. The test should stop when you come out of the position or 15 seconds has elapsed. This is your baseline balance. If you are able to balance for the full 15 seconds, try the one-legged stand test, as it is more challenging. If you are unable to balance at all in the tandem position, you can separate your feet slightly (four to six inches) to a near-tandem position and try the test. If you cannot perform this test, you may have poor balance and be at risk for falling during exercise, and you should consult your physician before proceeding with an exercise program. There are no norms for this test, but you can use it as a baseline for measuring your improvement. You can repeat this test after you've been exercising regularly; you should be able to increase the time you can stand in the tandem stance as you become more fit.

Establishing a Baseline of Mobility

Mobility, or gait, is a measure of how well you move around in your environment. It reflects how coordinated you are when you walk, how well you can move around obstacles, and how well you keep your balance while walking around turns. As we age, our gait is altered in a way that increases fall risk. Exercise has been shown to improve gait. The up-and-go test is a measure of mobility that you can use to establish a baseline for comparing yourself with age-related norms (Rikli and Jones 2001).

▷ *Up-and-Go*

The up-and-go test measures the time it takes you to rise from a chair, walk eight feet, turn around, and walk back to the chair and sit down. For this test, you will need a flat-backed stable chair, a measuring tape, a marker (pylon, beanbag, piece of colored tape), and a stopwatch. Place the chair against a wall for steadiness, then measure and mark a point 8 feet out from the chair. To start the test, sit in the middle of the chair with your back straight, your feet flat on the floor, and your knees in line with your feet. When you start the stopwatch, rise from the chair as fast as you can, walk quickly to the marker, turn around, and walk quickly back to the chair and sit down, then stop the watch. Write the time on your scorecard. This is your baseline mobility. Norms for healthy community-dwelling older adults are included in the appendix for comparison. Retest after you've been exercising regularly; you should be able to decrease the time it takes you to do the up-and-go.

Adjusting Exercise to Your Fitness Level

Depending on your starting fitness level, you'll want to adjust the starting point of your program either by reflecting on the amount of exercise you do regularly or according to the results of your fitness test. If you are completely or somewhat inactive or you score low on a fitness test, you should start your program at a low intensity level and progress slowly. You should also discuss your results and your intent to start an exercise program with your physician. If you are already an exerciser but have decided to incorporate some new exercises into your program, you should also start at a fairly low level but can progress more quickly if you respond well to the exercise. If you are already an exerciser or score well on a fitness test and want to improve further, you can start at a more moderate intensity and progress at a steady pace. If you score high on a given fitness test, you may want to add to your program to target other areas that may be weak. In chapter 6, we provide sample programs for

My Fitness Scorecard

	Baseline Date: _____	Follow-up 1 Date: _____	Follow-up 2 Date: _____
Aerobic fitness			
1.5-mile run Six-minute walk Two-minute step	Time: _____ Distance: _____ Steps: _____	Time: _____ Distance: _____ Steps: _____	Time: _____ Distance: _____ Steps: _____
Muscle strength			
1RM 6RM 10RM Sit-to-stand Arm curl	Pounds: _____ Pounds: _____ Pounds: _____ Stands: _____ Curls: _____	Pounds: _____ Pounds: _____ Pounds: _____ Stands: _____ Curls: _____	Pounds: _____ Pounds: _____ Pounds: _____ Stands: _____ Curls: _____
Flexibility			
Sit-and-reach Back scratch	Inches: _____ Inches: _____	Inches: _____ Inches: _____	Inches: _____ Inches: _____
Balance			
One-legged stand Tandem stance	Time: _____ Time: _____	Time: _____ Time: _____	Time: _____ Time: _____
Mobility			
Up-and-go	Time: _____	Time: _____	Time: _____

the beginning, or less fit, exerciser as well as for the intermediate and experienced, or more fit, exerciser.

Taking Safety Precautions

The risk of injury increases with any form of activity; however, the health risks associated with being inactive usually far outweigh the small risk of injury during exercise. If you have not already done so, you should inform your physician that you plan to begin an exercise program. You and your physician can discuss whether it is safe for you to start such a program, as well as any special concerns your physician may have. Along with your physician's advice, you should follow certain general safety guidelines when exercising. A few of these have already been discussed, such as including a warm-up and cool-down before and after your activity session and creating an emergency plan for how to deal with an injury if you are exercising alone. These tips along with other sound advice are listed in the sidebar below.

Tips for Safe Exercise

Include a warm-up and cool-down.

Exercise in a group or with a partner.

If you exercise alone, have a plan for what to do if you get hurt.

Wear proper clothing:

▸ Proper athletic shoes that fit

▸ Tops and pants or shorts made of breathable fabric

▸ A hat in sunny or cold weather

Stay hydrated!

In hot climates, exercise in an adequately ventilated room or at cooler times of the day.

Perform all exercises with proper form!

Don't push beyond your capabilities or exercise when you are ill.

You may wonder whether it is wise to exercise if you have been diagnosed with osteopenia or osteoporosis or if you have already suffered a fracture related to poor bone health. The answer almost unanimously is yes, unless your physician has advised you not to exercise. Exercise is known to improve bone health and prevent falls in women with osteopenia and osteoporosis, and it has been shown to restore strength, balance, and physical function in people who have suffered a fracture. Each case is discussed in slightly more detail in the following sections. An important consideration, however, is that the tolerance limits for exercise may be different for a woman with osteopenia versus a woman with osteoporosis versus a woman who has recently recovered from a hip fracture. For example, a healthy nonosteoporotic, postmenopausal woman may be able to engage in exercise at moderate to vigorous intensity, whereas a frail osteoporotic woman should exercise at low to moderate intensity and aim to maintain a level of physical function and reduce her fall risk. If you are unaccustomed to exercise, you should be supervised during the first few months of your program to ensure that you are doing the exercises correctly and at a safe level. If you engage in vigorous exercise programs or use heavy weight equipment, you will be safer in a supervised setting such as a group exercise class with a trained fitness leader or a health club with trained exercise professionals on site.

Exercising With Osteopenia

Exercise studies of women with low bone density are growing in number and show that women with osteopenia can exercise safely, even at moderate to high intensity, and that exercise may produce greater increases in bone density in women with osteopenia compared to those with normal or high bone density (Winters and Snow 2003). Generally, people who begin a training program with a low initial level of fitness experience greater benefit from training compared to those who are already fit. This finding likely holds true for women who are osteopenic and begin an exercise program directed at improving bone health. In fact, exercise should be a primary strategy for improving bone health in women with osteopenia because it is effective, inexpensive, and has additional health benefits.

Exercising With Osteoporosis

Although few in number, exercise studies of women who already have osteoporosis show that exercise can be performed with little risk of injury (e.g., fracture) and is quite beneficial. In my community exercise classes, a mildly osteoporotic participant performed our resistance exercise program without injury and was elated to find that the program and her medication helped significantly increase her bone density. We cannot say for sure how much of her improvement was due to exercise and how much to her medication, but she was able do the exercises without putting herself at risk for fracture, she enjoyed them, and they likely were of benefit to her bones and muscles. Other studies have had similar findings. Women with moderate to severe osteoporosis should be under the care of a physician and health care team (e.g., physical therapist) who can best judge the appropriate amount and type of activity for a given degree of disease.

If you have osteoporosis, exercise that lowers your risk of falling is an important strategy to incorporate into your action plan against fractures. We know that muscle weakness, poor balance, and difficulty walking increase the risk of falls. We have also shown through careful study that certain exercise programs can effectively combat these risk factors and prevent falls and fall-related injuries. These studies were summarized briefly in chapter 4 and provide the basis for the fall-prevention exercises outlined in chapter 6.

Currently, there is no estimate of the amount of exercise women with osteoporosis can tolerate without fracture. Your activity limitations should be discussed with your physician and physical therapist. Obviously, the more severe your osteoporosis, the more care you must take to avoid putting too much force on your bones. Practical and conservative recommendations suggest that some movements should be avoided, and these are listed in the sidebar on page 60.

Exercises and Movements to Avoid If You Have Osteoporosis

Very high impact exercise (e.g., jumping with added weight)

Back flexion against resistance (e.g., lifting your back off the floor from a lying position with an object in your arms, such as a child; sit-ups against resistance)

Lifting loads overhead (e.g., lifting a heavy box off a high shelf)

Lifting heavy objects some distance away from your body (e.g., bending over to get a turkey out of the oven or to pick up a grandchild)

Quick twisting movements (e.g., golf swing)

Exercising After a Fracture

Fracture is an unfortunate consequence of osteoporosis but does not preclude you from exercising again. Bone pain is common in the weeks following fracture, and injury to the muscles and ligaments may result in additional discomfort for extended periods. Depending on the location and severity of a fracture, it can lead to severe reductions in mobility and function, which in turn lead to loss of independence and possibly depression. Activity levels are always curtailed after a fracture to allow for recovery, and this period of inactivity can be fairly long if the fracture requires surgery. Inactivity can lead to a loss of physical conditioning, strength, and function. People who suffer a fracture resulting from a fall are often hesitant to resume exercise because they are fearful of falling again. These consequences of a fracture can all be addressed through physical rehabilitation and exercise. Some studies even suggest that certain back-strengthening exercises can protect against the risk of a spine fracture, but this proposition is beyond the scope of this text and should be discussed with one's health care team (Pfeifer et al. 2004).

Following surgery or the initial recovery period, physical therapy is necessary to restore basic mobility and should continue until one is able to move relatively pain free. Once mobility is restored, a limited program of regular exercise that progresses according to one's tolerance and capabilities can begin. This program should aim to restore aerobic fitness (functional ability) for general health and to restore and improve muscle strength and balance for fall risk reduction. This program should be developed with the guidance of a physical therapist, who can best assess a safe starting level and progression of exercise.

Summary

Establishing your baseline level of fitness is helpful in judging the appropriate starting level for your exercise program and provides you with a way of measuring your progress. Several types of tests can help you evaluate your starting fitness level in different areas. Choose a test that is most appropriate for you given your resources, physical abilities, and confidence level. Do not perform a test unless you can establish a safe environment and are confident you can perform the test with minimal risk of injury. Consider having a family member or friend available to assist you during any test, particularly if you are less fit. Evaluating your baseline fitness is not necessary when beginning an exercise program but can be a useful addition. If you perform the tests, keep track of your performance on a scorecard and use this information to identify your strengths and weaknesses as well as to determine an appropriate starting level for your exercise program. Repeat the tests after you've been exercising regularly (in two to three months) so you can see your improvements. Seeing an improvement in your performance can be a strong motivator to keep going!

ACTION PLAN:
EVALUATING YOUR BASELINE FITNESS

- ☐ Establish your baseline fitness level and set your program accordingly.
- ☐ Use your baseline to chart your progress during exercise training.
- ☐ Know the safety precautions to consider during exercise.
- ☐ Don't avoid exercise if you have osteopenia, osteoporosis, or have experienced a fracture. Exercise is an important part of your rehabilitation plan and should be developed in conjunction with your health care team.

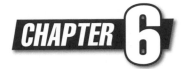
CREATING A CUSTOMIZED EXERCISE PLAN

We're finally ready to get down to the business of developing an exercise plan! The first five chapters have given you a foundation of knowledge about osteoporosis, falls, exercise training, and the type and amount of exercise that will best lower your risk of fracture. You are a virtual expert at this point! Now we need to put all of this knowledge to work in creating a "prescription" for optimizing your bone health. This prescription is not unlike a prescription you'd receive from your doctor telling you exactly what drug to take, how much of it to take, and how often and how long to take it. When your medication runs out, you must check back in with your doctor, who reassesses your symptoms and either renews your prescription, makes adjustments, switches to a different drug, or has you stop altogether. The difference between your exercise prescription and one your doctor might give you for medication is that your exercise program is intended to continue indefinitely and *you* are in charge of your prescription. Ultimately, you have to set the goals for your program, design the program to meet those goals, and make adjustments to your program to accommodate changes in your goals, your fitness, or your preferences over time.

In this chapter, we'll discuss how to set goals for your exercise program and how to design a program that will meet those goals. I'll also provide several sample programs that can be used as models in designing one of your own. You can choose to follow one of these programs or use bits and pieces of them that best fit your likes and needs. Or you could design a completely new program for yourself based on what you've learned in this book. In the next chapter, I'll give you clear instructions and illustrations on how to perform the specific exercises discussed in this chapter safely and effectively. My goal is to provide you with the tools you need to build a lifelong program for avoiding a fracture to optimize your long-term health.

Preparing to Exercise

If you are a beginning exerciser, you would be wise to obtain a physician's clearance. Since it is impossible to determine whether you can safely begin exercising, I recommend discussing your intention to exercise with your physician or other primary health care provider. This will give your health care provider an opportunity to be sure there are no known or suspected conditions that would preclude you from exercising so you can proceed with less risk of injury. The risk of an adverse exercise-related event is greatest during vigorous exercise. Thus, if you are a new exerciser, you can minimize your risk of injury by starting at a low intensity and progressing gradually.

If you plan to begin an exercise program or are already a beginning exerciser and want to progress to a moderate-intensity program, you should fill out the Physical Activity Readiness Questionnaire (PAR-Q) to help you decide whether you need to see your physician before starting such a program (see figure 6.1). The PAR-Q was specifically designed to screen individuals wishing to participate in a moderate-intensity exercise program for issues such as underlying cardiac or bone and joint problems that might cause an adverse exercise-related event. If you answer yes to any question on the PAR-Q, you should see your health care provider prior to beginning a moderate-intensity program. You may also benefit from participation in a *professionally guided* pre-exercise assessment and prescription (ACSM 2005). If you answer no to all questions but are currently ill or not feeling well, you should delay exercise until you have completely recovered.

If you are a current exerciser and intend to progress to a more vigorous intensity program, you are urged to consult with your health care provider to make sure there are no reasons why you should not participate in such a program.

Setting Goals for Your Program

Any lifestyle change you make, including exercise, should be undertaken with a goal in mind. When you invest money in your child's college fund, you choose an investment strategy that gives you a good return without too much risk. You check your monthly statements to make sure your investments are paying off as expected. If they are doing well, you consider going after a bigger payoff. If they are doing poorly, you change your strategy. If they are doing just as expected, you stick with your plan. You should track your investment in your exercise program as diligently as you would your child's education money. The first step is to set goals for

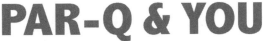

PAR-Q & YOU

(A Questionnaire for People Aged 15 to 69)

Regular physical activity is fun and healthy, and increasingly more people are starting to become more active every day. Being more active is very safe for most people. However, some people should check with their doctor before they start becoming much more physically active.

If you are planning to become much more physically active than you are now, start by answering the seven questions in the box below. If you are between the ages of 15 and 69, the PAR-Q will tell you if you should check with your doctor before you start. If you are over 69 years of age, and you are not used to being very active, check with your doctor.

Common sense is your best guide when you answer these questions. Please read the questions carefully and answer each one honestly: check YES or NO.

YES	NO		
☐	☐	1.	**Has your doctor ever said that you have a heart condition <u>and</u> that you should only do physical activity recommended by a doctor?**
☐	☐	2.	**Do you feel pain in your chest when you do physical activity?**
☐	☐	3.	**In the past month, have you had chest pain when you were not doing physical activity?**
☐	☐	4.	**Do you lose your balance because of dizziness or do you ever lose consciousness?**
☐	☐	5.	**Do you have a bone or joint problem (for example, back, knee or hip) that could be made worse by a change in your physical activity?**
☐	☐	6.	**Is your doctor currently prescribing drugs (for example, water pills) for your blood pressure or heart condition?**
☐	☐	7.	**Do you know of <u>any other reason</u> why you should not do physical activity?**

If

you

answered

YES to one or more questions

Talk with your doctor by phone or in person BEFORE you start becoming much more physically active or BEFORE you have a fitness appraisal. Tell your doctor about the PAR-Q and which questions you answered YES.

- You may be able to do any activity you want — as long as you start slowly and build up gradually. Or, you may need to restrict your activities to those which are safe for you. Talk with your doctor about the kinds of activities you wish to participate in and follow his/her advice.
- Find out which community programs are safe and helpful for you.

NO to all questions

If you answered NO honestly to <u>all</u> PAR-Q questions, you can be reasonably sure that you can:
- start becoming much more physically active – begin slowly and build up gradually. This is the safest and easiest way to go.
- take part in a fitness appraisal – this is an excellent way to determine your basic fitness so that you can plan the best way for you to live actively. It is also highly recommended that you have your blood pressure evaluated. If your reading is over 144/94, talk with your doctor before you start becoming much more physically active.

DELAY BECOMING MUCH MORE ACTIVE:
- if you are not feeling well because of a temporary illness such as a cold or a fever – wait until you feel better; or
- if you are or may be pregnant – talk to your doctor before you start becoming more active.

PLEASE NOTE: If your health changes so that you then answer YES to any of the above questions, tell your fitness or health professional. Ask whether you should change your physical activity plan.

<u>Informed Use of the PAR-Q:</u> The Canadian Society for Exercise Physiology, Health Canada, and their agents assume no liability for persons who undertake physical activity, and if in doubt after completing this questionnaire, consult your doctor prior to physical activity.

No changes permitted. You are encouraged to photocopy the PAR-Q but only if you use the entire form.

NOTE: If the PAR-Q is being given to a person before he or she participates in a physical activity program or a fitness appraisal, this section may be used for legal or administrative purposes.

"I have read, understood and completed this questionnaire. Any questions I had were answered to my full satisfaction."

NAME _____

SIGNATURE _____ DATE _____

SIGNATURE OF PARENT _____ WITNESS _____
or GUARDIAN (for participants under the age of majority)

Note: This physical activity clearance is valid for a maximum of 12 months from the date it is completed and becomes invalid if your condition changes so that you would answer YES to any of the seven questions.

CSEP
SCPE © Canadian Society for Exercise Physiology   Supported by: 🍁 Health   Santé
                                                                      Canada   Canada   continued on other side...

Figure 6.1   Physical Activity Readiness Questionnaire.

From *Action Plan for Osteoporosis* by Kerri Winters-Stone, © 2005 American College of Sports Medicine, Champaign, IL: Human Kinetics.
Source: Physical Activity Readiness Questionnaire (PAR-Q) © 2002. Reprinted with permission from the Canadian Society for Exercise Physiology. http://www.csep.ca/forms.asp

PAR-Q & YOU

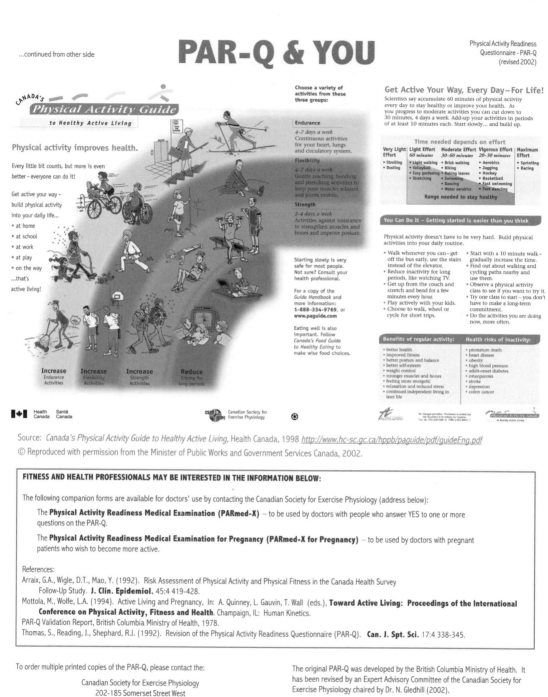

Source: *Canada's Physical Activity Guide to Healthy Active Living*, Health Canada, 1998 http://www.hc-sc.gc.ca/hppb/paguide/pdf/guideEng.pdf
© Reproduced with permission from the Minister of Public Works and Government Services Canada, 2002.

FITNESS AND HEALTH PROFESSIONALS MAY BE INTERESTED IN THE INFORMATION BELOW:

The following companion forms are available for doctors' use by contacting the Canadian Society for Exercise Physiology (address below):

The **Physical Activity Readiness Medical Examination (PARmed-X)** – to be used by doctors with people who answer YES to one or more questions on the PAR-Q.

The **Physical Activity Readiness Medical Examination for Pregnancy (PARmed-X for Pregnancy)** – to be used by doctors with pregnant patients who wish to become more active.

References:
Arraix, G.A., Wigle, D.T., Mao, Y. (1992). Risk Assessment of Physical Activity and Physical Fitness in the Canada Health Survey
    Follow-Up Study. **J. Clin. Epidemiol.** 45:4 419-428.
Mottola, M., Wolfe, L.A. (1994). Active Living and Pregnancy, In: A. Quinney, L. Gauvin, T. Wall (eds.), **Toward Active Living: Proceedings of the International
    Conference on Physical Activity, Fitness and Health**. Champaign, IL: Human Kinetics.
PAR-Q Validation Report, British Columbia Ministry of Health, 1978.
Thomas, S., Reading, J., Shephard, R.J. (1992). Revision of the Physical Activity Readiness Questionnaire (PAR-Q). **Can. J. Spt. Sci.** 17:4 338-345.

To order multiple printed copies of the PAR-Q, please contact the:

Canadian Society for Exercise Physiology
202-185 Somerset Street West
Ottawa, ON K2P 0J2
Tel. 1-877-651-3755 • FAX (613) 234-3565
Online: www.csep.ca

The original PAR-Q was developed by the British Columbia Ministry of Health. It has been revised by an Expert Advisory Committee of the Canadian Society for Exercise Physiology chaired by Dr. N. Gledhill (2002).

Disponible en français sous le titre «Questionnaire sur l'aptitude à l'activité physique - Q-AAP (revisé 2002)».

© Canadian Society for Exercise Physiology

Supported by: Health Canada Santé Canada

Figure 6.1 *(continued)*
From *Action Plan for Osteoporosis* by Kerri Winters-Stone, © 2005 American College of Sports Medicine, Champaign, IL: Human Kinetics.

your exercise investment so that your time and effort pay off. The next step is to choose the right exercise strategy to meet your goals, knowing that you will need to assess your progress from time to time to make sure your strategy is working and make any necessary adjustments.

Goal setting is important for the reasons already stated as well as several others, including the following:

- Setting goals gives you direction by giving you a specific objective to strive for.
- Setting goals helps motivate you to exercise regularly.
- Reaching your goals gives you a sense of accomplishment, and you deserve to be rewarded for your hard work!

How to Set Goals

Goal setting is more art than science, but following some general guidelines can be helpful. Goals need to be realistic so that you set yourself up for success rather than failure. At the same time, goals need to be challenging so that you push yourself enough to see improvements. You should set both short- and long-term goals that give you both an immediate objective to strive for as well as a broader, overall objective for your program. Goals need to be continually revisited so that if they are too lofty, too shortsighted, or have changed focus, you can revise them accordingly. Here are some examples of goal setting.

- *Alice* is a 58-year-old postmenopausal woman with mild osteopenia and a family history of osteoporosis. She lost 2 percent of her hip bone mass over the past year. Her mother suffered a hip fracture at age 75. Alice is worried about her risk of a hip fracture and wants to start an exercise program to reduce that risk. She currently walks three times per week but knows she must do more to prevent further bone loss. She loves her walking program and doesn't want to give it up. You work with her in setting her short- and long-term goals and have decided on the following:

Short-term goal: Add jumping exercise to her walking routine by working up to 50 jumps, three times per week, over the next three months. (Alice would assess her program after three months and then set another short-term goal, which might be to work up to 100 jumps, three times per week, over the subsequent three months.)

Long-term goal: Maintain bone mass of her hip by engaging in regular bone-building exercise and other bone-healthy habits.

- *Earl* is a 75-year-old man with osteoporosis at the spine and hip. He has fallen twice in the past year. He is currently taking medication to improve his bone mass but wants to further reduce his risk of fracture by preventing future falls. He did a self-assessment and found that he scored low on leg strength (in the sit-to-stand test) and on mobility (in the up-and-go test). He works with you to set the following short- and long-term goals for his exercise program:

> Short-term goal: To begin a strength and balance training program that would improve leg strength by increasing sit-to-stand performance by three stands in three months and would improve mobility by increasing up-and-go time by one second in three months.

> Long-term goal: To prevent future falls and lower fracture risk by engaging in regular exercise and other fall-prevention habits.

Short- and Long-Term Goals

As you can see from the previous examples, short- and long-term goals have distinct features, but both give you something to shoot for. Short-term goals need to be realistic, achievable, and measurable. They are what you will use to determine if your exercise program is meeting your needs and, if it isn't, what adjustments you need to make. You may want to set conservative goals at first because the last thing you want to do is to set a goal that you can never achieve. There is nothing like failure to motivate you to quit exercising. In contrast, success will motivate you to keep at it! Your short-term goals need to be set with your starting fitness and activity levels in mind as well, so that the program is neither too hard nor too easy. Long-term goals should reflect the reason you are exercising in the first place. These goals may be hard to measure in the short run. For example, if your ultimate goal is to prevent a fracture, you will only know that you've met your goal if you never have another fracture. It is hard to measure your success in terms of something that does not occur. This underscores the importance of setting short-term, measurable goals, but long-term goals are still needed to give your program an overall sense of purpose.

Writing Your Exercise Prescription

Now that you've set your goals, the next step is to create the right prescription for reaching them. We will apply what you learned in chapters 4 and 5 to design an appropriate program based on your starting fitness level and goals. I'll give you many options to choose from when putting your program together so that you can find what fits best for you and your lifestyle. I'll also show you how to progress your program so that it continues to be challenging and effective.

The basic program descriptions are organized by exercise type. As you learned in chapter 4, moderate- to vigorous-intensity programs of aerobic, resistance, or impact exercise can increase or maintain bone mass. Moderate-intensity resistance training plus a few simple balance exercises can help prevent falls. Combining several types of exercise in your exercise plan can also be a comprehensive way to improve your bone health *and* reduce your fall risk. Several sample programs will be included throughout the chapter so you can use them as models for your program. Chapter 7 provides specific descriptions and illustrations of the exercises used in the sample programs.

Stages of Progression

Three stages of training are used in setting the appropriate amount of exercise for your program and in shaping your long-term plan: the initial conditioning stage, the improvement stage, and the maintenance stage. These stages, which are described in the following sections, provide the framework for how to move through your exercise plan over the long term. A lifetime exercise plan usually progresses through each of these stages in succession. We will refer to these stages when outlining the starting point of your exercise program.

Initial Conditioning Stage

The initial conditioning stage is sometimes referred to as the "familiarization" stage because the goal is simply to get you used to doing a new type of activity. During this first stage, you want to avoid exercising too intensely or you may risk getting injured or getting turned off to the program because it is too hard. As you move through the initial stage, you should gradually increase the amount of time (duration) you exercise so that you adapt to doing more of a particular activity. The initial conditioning stage lasts about four to eight weeks, depending on your progress. All beginning exercisers should start at the initial stage. More experienced exercisers may want to start at the initial stage if they are doing exercises that are new to them, or they may choose to move right into the improvement stage. For example, a regular walker who has never done resistance exercise may choose to start in the initial stage of a resistance training program but may find that she's ready to move to the improvement stage rather quickly. If you have never exercised before, you may want to begin with a simple walking program for the first few months. I've listed a beginning walking program in table 6.1 that will help you become more physically active safely so that you can build the confidence to try exercise that is a little more challenging than walking.

Improvement Stage

The improvement stage is where you should start to notice some physical changes because you'll be exercising a little more vigorously. During this stage, you'll gradually increase the overload of your program by increasing the intensity, time, and frequency, one at a time. The improvement stage

Table 6.1   Beginner Walking Program

Weeks	Program
1-2	Walk 10-15 minutes at a slow but steady pace.
3-4	Add 2-4 minutes to your daily walk over 2 weeks.
5-6	Add 2-4 minutes to your daily walk over 2 weeks.
7-8	Add 2-4 minutes to your daily walk over 2 weeks.
9-10	Walk a little more briskly.
11-12	Enjoy your accomplishment and consider moving to the progression phase of exercise if you tolerated weeks 9-10 well; if you are having difficulty with this program, consult your physician and seek guidance from an exercise professional.

typically lasts about four to six months, depending on your progress. If you are satisfied with your progress at the end of this stage, then move on to the maintenance stage. Depending on your goal, you may want to see further improvement, so you can extend the improvement stage by increasing the overload again.

Maintenance Stage

The maintenance stage is the ultimate goal of your program. Once you have achieved the goals you set for the improvement stage, the next step is to maintain your program for a lifetime. Remember our earlier discussion on the "use it or lose it" principle in chapter 3? We know from research that the benefits you gain from exercise are lost if you stop being active on a regular basis. When you get to the maintenance stage, you can slightly decrease the amount of exercise you do because you are no longer pushing to change your body. For example, you can decrease the intensity or duration of exercise by a small amount. Or if you are happy with things as they are, you can keep plugging along as you have been. You now view exercise as a lifelong proposition, and you want to prevent injury and boredom. Thus, the maintenance stage is the perfect time to try some new activities. Instead of going to aerobics class one day, try a yoga class. Or instead of doing your lower body exercises at home, go for a hike on a course that includes some hills. Perhaps you even feel fit enough to run in a local race. You might also add a new type of exercise that challenges another aspect of your fitness. By this stage, you are officially an experienced exerciser—a virtual amateur athlete—and can venture into new territory with confidence.

Adding Aerobic Exercise

Moderate to vigorous aerobic exercise can improve or maintain bone mass of the hip and spine and has additional benefits as outlined in chapter 4. This type of exercise program would be most suited for people who have osteopenia or mild osteoporosis and want to improve their bone mass or to prevent or slow further bone loss. For women with advanced osteoporosis or those who have had a recent fracture, this type of program is probably too rigorous unless physician approval is obtained. In these women, maintaining a regular exercise program that includes fall-prevention exercises would be appropriate.

To challenge the skeleton, the aerobic exercise chosen should be weight bearing, although rowing exercise may be of particular benefit to the spine. Examples of weight-bearing aerobic exercises are listed in table 6.2, and a few of these are illustrated in chapter 7. These aerobic exercises are categorized according to their intensity level so that you can choose the type of activity that best matches your initial fitness level and your goals.

Table 6.2 Weight-Bearing Aerobic Activities

Moderate level	Vigorous level
Low-impact aerobics	High-impact aerobics (step class)
Moderate-paced dancing (waltz)	Fast-paced dancing (salsa, jitterbug, disco)
Brisk walking (3-4.5 mph)	Fast/race walking (5 mph or faster) and jogging/running
Brisk hiking on level ground	Brisk hiking or hiking up hills
Tennis: Doubles	Tennis: Singles
Light rowing (machine or boat)	Fast rowing (machine or boat)

The general exercise prescription for aerobic exercise aimed at improving bone health is to reach a *minimum* target of 30 minutes of continuous moderate-intensity exercise, five days per week, similar to the general public health recommendations for physical activity (Pate et al. 1995). Remember that walking exercise may need to be done at a vigorous pace in order to improve bone health. To see greater improvement, you can increase the amount of exercise you do by increasing the intensity, duration, or frequency of exercise. Generally, the upper range for effective aerobic exercise is 60 minutes of vigorous-intensity exercise, five to seven days per week. Any more than this and you may risk injury or burnout.

Gauging Intensity

As discussed earlier, there are several ways to determine how much effort you are putting forth during exercise (intensity), which in turn will tell you whether you are working too hard or not hard enough. The methods we will use are the heart rate reserve (HRR) method and the Rating of Perceived Exertion (RPE) scale. You may have seen posters in health clubs or community centers that show your "target heart rate range."

Heart rate reserve method (HRR). The HRR method has you gauge your effort by monitoring your heart rate from time to time during exercise. This method is fairly precise and gives you a clear idea of whether you are at the right intensity. It may be especially useful for beginning exercisers who aren't exactly sure how they should be feeling when they are in the right intensity range. Guidelines for determining your HRR and a sample calculation appear in the sidebar below. The HRR ranges for low-, moderate-, and vigorous-intensity exercise are listed in table 6.3. Table 6.4 gives a general grid for HRR based on HRmax and resting heart rate. Instructions on how to take your heart rate during exercise can be found in the sidebar on page 74.

Calculating Your HRR

Use this formula to calculate your heart rate reserve:

Moderate target heart rate range = ([HRmax – HRrest] × 0.40-0.59)
Vigorous target heart rate range = ([HRmax – HRrest] × 0.60-0.85)

where HRmax equals your estimated age-predicted maximal heart rate based on the formula 220 – age and HRrest equals your estimated resting heart rate, which is determined shortly after waking or after resting quietly for 10 to 15 minutes.

Table 6.3   Heart Rate Ranges

HRR range	Intensity
20-39% HRR	Low
40-59% HRR	Moderate
60-84% HRR	Vigorous

Who should NOT use the HRR method? Individuals who are taking medications known to alter their heart rate response to exercise should not use this method. For example, people with certain heart conditions are

Table 6.4   Training Heart Rates*

	HR$_{max}$ method		Resting heart rate					
			60 beats per min.		70 beats per min.		80 beats per min.	
			Heart rate reserve method					
HR$_{max}$ (beats per min.)	70%	85%	60%	80%	60%	80%	60%	80%
140	98	119	108	124	112	126	116	128
150	105	128	114	132	118	134	122	136
160	112	136	120	140	124	142	128	144
170	119	145	126	148	130	150	134	152
180	126	153	132	156	136	158	140	160
190	133	162	138	164	142	166	146	168
200	140	170	144	172	148	174	152	176

*Calculated for age adjusted estimates of maximal heart rates for 20- to 80-year-olds (220 − age) using both the percent of maximal hearet rate and the heart rate reserve methods, with three different resting heart rates (60, 70, 80 beats per minute) used in the latter calculation.

Adapted, by permission, from American College of Sports Medicine (ACSM), 2000, *ACSM's guidelines for exercise testing and prescription*, 6th edition (Baltimore: Lippincott Williams & Wilkins), 149.

put on medications that slow their heart rate when at rest and during exercise. If they were to use the HRR method as a guide in judging exercise intensity, they would likely find that their heart rate does not reach the target range, even though they feel they are putting forth a lot of effort. Because the medication artificially lowers their heart rate, increasing intensity to reach the HRR target range would put them at too hard a pace and could be dangerous.

The RPE method.   The RPE scale for judging intensity has you self-rate the level of effort you put forth during exercise according to a set scale. The scale ranges from 6 to 20, with 6 being the lowest level of effort (i.e., resting) and 20 the highest (i.e., sprinting at full speed). Figure 6.3 shows the RPE scale and the corresponding effort ratings. If you are unaccustomed to exercise, you may have difficulty matching your effort to the right rating. In this case, you could use both the HRR method and the RPE method to learn what various levels of effort (measured by HRR) make your body feel like (measured by RPE). If you use the RPE scale, you must be honest. Figure 6.3 lists the RPE ranges for exercises of varying intensities. Light exercise (9-11) corresponds to low-intensity exercise, somewhat hard

Taking Your Heart Rate (Pulse)

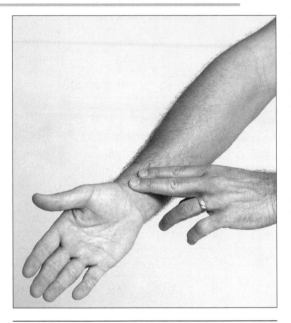

Figure 6.2 Taking pulse at the wrist.

The recommended method for taking your heart rate is to count the pulses you feel on your radial artery (located on your wrist in line with the base of your thumb). Place the tips of your index and middle fingers (not the thumb, which has a pulse of its own) over the artery and apply light pressure until you feel a pulse (see figure 6.2). Using a stopwatch or a watch with a second hand, count the number of pulses over a 30-second period and multiply by two to obtain your heart rate in beats per minute. During exercise, you will need to shorten the length of time that you count pulses to 10 or 15 seconds and multiply by six (for a 10-second count) or four (for a 15-second count), respectively, to get your exercise heart rate in beats per minute.

(12-14) corresponds to moderate-intensity exercise, and hard to extremely hard (15-19) corresponds to vigorous-intensity exercise.

Beginner Aerobic Exercise Program

If you have never exercised before and are in the initial conditioning stage, you should begin with lower level aerobic exercises and work up to the more challenging exercises listed in table 6.2. A sample four-week aerobic exercise program for someone in the initial stage of training may look like that in table 6.5.

To progress to the improvement stage, you would increase the intensity of your program over the next month or two. After adjusting to this intensity, you could exercise

6	No exertion at all
7	Extremely light
8	
9	Very light
10	
11	Light
12	
13	Somewhat hard
14	
15	Hard (heavy)
16	
17	Very hard
18	
19	Extremely hard
20	Maximal exertion

Borg RPE scale
© Gunnar Borg, 1970, 1985, 1994, 1998

Figure 6.3 The Borg RPE scale.
G. Borg, 1998, *Borg's perceived exertion and pain scales* (Champaign, IL: Human Kinetics), 47.

Table 6.5   Beginner Aerobic Exercise Program

Monday	Tuesday	Wednesday	Thursday	Friday	Saturday	Sunday	Program change
Week 1							
Walk 15-20 min at 40-50% HRR or 11-12 RPE	Off or stretch	Bench stepping for 15-20 min at 40-50% HRR or 11-12 RPE	Off or stretch	Walk 15-20 min at 40-50% HRR or 11-12 RPE	Off or stretch	Leisure or non-weight-bearing activity (gardening, swimming)	*None*
Week 2							
Walk 20-25 min at 40-50% HRR or 11-12 RPE	Off or stretch	Bench stepping for 20-25 min at 40-50% HRR or 11-12 RPE	Off or stretch	Walk 20-25 min at 40-50% HRR or 11-12 RPE	Off or stretch	Leisure or non-weight-bearing activity (gardening, swimming)	*Increased time by 5 min per session*
Week 3							
Walk/jog 20-25 min at 45-55% HRR or 12-13 RPE	Off or stretch	Bench stepping (faster) for 20-25 min at 50-60% HRR or 12-13 RPE	Off or stretch	Walk/jog 20-25 min at 50-60% HRR or 12-13 RPE	Off or stretch	Leisure or non-weight-bearing activity (gardening, swimming)	*Increased intensity by 5% HRR or 1 RPE*
Week 4							
Walk/jog 25-30 min at 45-55% HRR or 12-13 RPE	Off or stretch	Bench stepping (faster) for 25-30 min at 45-55% HRR or 12-13 RPE	Off or stretch	Walk/jog 25-30 min at 45-55% HRR or 12-13 RPE	Off or stretch	Bench stepping (faster) for 25-30 min at 45-55% HRR or 12-13 RPE	*Increased time by 5 min per session*

Every exercise session would include a 5- to 10-minute warm-up before exercise and a 5- to 10-minute cool-down after exercise. Exercises listed as moderate in Table 6.2 could be substituted for the walking or bench stepping listed in this sample program.

a little longer each session for the next few months and then add another day after that. A progression scale might look like this:

Month	Progression
2-4	Increase intensity by 5 percent HRR or 1 RPE (could move from a walk/jog to a jog) over weeks 1-2 of each month.
	Increase duration by five minutes per session over weeks 3-4 of each month.
5	Add another day per week of aerobic exercise (increase from three to four days per week).
6	Move into maintenance phase or begin another progression cycle.

Intermediate Aerobic Exercise Program

If you've already been exercising at a low to moderate intensity of aerobic exercise and want to progress to a more rigorous program, you could start by increasing the intensity of your workouts, then the duration, then the frequency, as in the previous progression scale. For example, if Jennifer already attends two low-impact aerobics classes per week but wants to move to a more rigorous program that will help increase her bone mass, she may want to follow the sample 12-week program outlined in table 6.6.

To progress to the maintenance phase, she could increase the intensity of her program over the next month or two. After adjusting to this intensity, she could exercise a little longer each session for the next few months and then add another day after that. The first few months of a

Table 6.6   Intermediate Aerobic Exercise Program

Monday	Tuesday	Wednesday	Thursday	Friday	Saturday	Sunday	Program change
Weeks 1-3							
Aerobics class for 25-30 min at 60-70% HRR or 14-15 RPE	Off or stretch	Jogging or cardio-vascular machine(s) at gym* for 25-30 min at 60-70% HRR or 14-15 RPE	Off or stretch	Aerobics class for 25-30 min at 60-70% HRR or 14-15 RPE	Off or stretch	Leisure or sport activity; could be non-weight bearing	*Increased intensity of aerobic exercise*

Monday	Tuesday	Wednesday	Thursday	Friday	Saturday	Sunday	*Program change*
Weeks 4-6							
Jogging or cardio-vascular machine(s) at gym* for 30-35 min at 60-70% HRR or 14-15 RPE	Off or stretch	Aerobics class for 30-35 min at 60-70% HRR or 14-15 RPE	Off or stretch	Jogging or cardio-vascular machine(s) at gym* for 30-35 min at 60-70% HRR or 14-15 RPE	Off or stretch	Leisurely activity or sport activity; could be non-weight bearing	*Increased time by 5 min per session*
Weeks 7-9							
Aerobics class for 30-35 min at 65-75% HRR or 15-16 RPE	Off or stretch	Jogging or cardio-vascular machine(s) at gym* for 30-35 min at 65-75% HRR or 15-16 RPE	Off or stretch	Aerobics class for 30-35 min at 65-75% HRR or 15-16 RPE	Off or stretch	Leisure or sport activity; could be non-weight bearing	*Increased intensity of aerobic exercise by 5% HRR or 1-2 RPE*
Weeks 10-12							
Jogging or cardio-vascular machine(s) at gym* for 30-35 min at 65-75% HRR or 15-16 RPE	Off or stretch	Aerobics class for 30-35 min at 65-75% HRR or 15-16 RPE	Off or stretch	Jogging or cardio-vascular machine(s) at gym* for 30-35 min at 65-75% HRR or 15-16 RPE	Aerobics class for 30-35 min at 65-75% HRR or 15-16 RPE	Leisure or sport activity; could be non-weight bearing	*Added another day of exercise*

*Cardiovascular machines at gym that target bone: rowing, stair climbing, treadmill.

Every exercise session would include a 5- to 10-minute warm-up before exercise and a 5- to 10-minute cool-down after exercise.

maintenance stage for the intermediate program described earlier might look like this:

Month	Program change
1	Decrease duration of exercise by five minutes per session.
2	Decrease intensity by 5 percent of HRR or 1 RPE.
3	Substitute one day per week with new activity.
4+	Maintain program at this level.

Adding Resistance Exercise

Moderate to vigorous resistance exercise can improve or maintain bone mass of the hip and spine and is key in preventing falls. Resistance training also has additional benefits as outlined in chapter 4. This type of exercise program would be most suited for people who have osteopenia and want to improve their bone mass and for those with osteoporosis who want to prevent further bone loss and particularly to prevent falls. Since resistance exercise is key for fall prevention, people who have already experienced a fracture may be able to engage in a program of light- to moderate-intensity resistance exercise, with physician clearance and consultation with a physical therapist. Starting out with an *intense* resistance exercise program is too rigorous for women with advanced osteoporosis or those who have had a recent fracture.

To challenge the skeleton, the resistance exercise chosen should be weight bearing and should target muscle groups attached to the hip and spine (see "Specificity of Resistance Training"). Examples of effective resistance exercises and illustrations of them are given in chapter 7.

Specificity of Resistance Training

One of the advantages of resistance training is that you can target almost any one muscle, large or small, with a given exercise. Technically, you could focus on strengthening the biceps only by performing exercise that specifically targets that muscle. Or you could focus on an entire muscle group, such as the back muscles. So which muscles do you target to improve bone mass at the spine? At the hip? At both sites? Which muscles do you target to prevent falls? If you remember the principle of specificity, you can determine which muscles need to be trained to achieve the desired effect. For example, if the goal is to improve spine bone mass, the exercises should work the upper body. If the goal is to improve hip bone mass, the exercises should work the lower body. Similarly, if the goal is to prevent falls, you should work the leg muscles that will improve balance and help you recover from a trip, slip, or stumble. I'll try to simplify resistance training for you by categorizing the exercises into upper and lower body workouts in chapter 7.

Gauging Intensity

We will use a couple of methods to determine intensity for resistance training: the repetition maximum method and the RPE scale described previously. Guidelines for determining your repetition maximum and a sample calculation appear in the sidebar below. The RM and RPE ranges for low-, moderate-, and vigorous-intensity exercises are listed in table 6.7.

Table 6.7   Repetition Maximum and Rating of Perceived Exertion Ranges

RM	RPE	Intensity
13-20	10-11	Low
8-12	12-14	Moderate
1-7	15-17	Vigorous (high)

Determining Your Repetition Maximum

Knowing how much weight to lift is more trial and error than precise science. Because each of us comes to a resistance training program with different levels of muscle strength, a weight that may be difficult for one person to lift may not be very challenging for another. One way to determine how much weight you should lift is by determining your repetition maximum, or RM. Your RM is the amount of weight you can lift a given number of times and no more. For example, if I can only do 10 biceps curls with a 15-pound weight and cannot lift it an 11th time, then 15 pounds is my 10RM for the biceps curl. The weight for a given RM will also differ for different movements. For example, although my 10RM for the biceps curl is 15 pounds, my 10RM for the leg press will likely be much higher because I have much more muscle in my legs than in my arms. My 10RM weight for the leg press is probably closer to 100 pounds. Determining the right RM weight for you and for each exercise will require some guesswork. Of course, the best option is to get help from a personal trainer or fitness professional, but if you don't have access to professional advice these guidelines will help you estimate the correct weight. To avoid injury, it is better to guess on the lighter side than on the heavier side. In trying to find my 10RM weight for the biceps curl, I might pick up a 12-pound weight and see if I could lift it 11 times. If I could, I would stop and pick up a 15-pound weight and see if I could lift it no more than 10 times. If I could lift it anywhere between 8 and 10 times and no more, I'd stick with that weight. If the first attempt with the 12-pound weight was too hard, I'd drop down to a 10-pound weight and try for 10 reps again. As you can see, the first time you try to determine your RM weights, you may get quite a workout. But once you get a feel for what weight is right for you for each exercise, you'll be ready to start training. Remember, though, that as you adapt to resistance training, you should be able to lift your RM weight a few more times than in your original set because you are getting stronger. Once that happens, you are ready to increase your weight, back off a couple of repetitions, and start working your way back up again. This is the essence of overload for resistance exercise!

Beginner Resistance Program to Improve Bone Health

If you have never exercised before and are in the initial conditioning stage, you should begin with lower level resistance exercises aimed at building a base of muscle endurance and work up to more challenging exercises that will build strength. The focus of this initial program is to get used to doing regular resistance training and to do so safely and effectively. To do this, the resistance training should consist of lifting moderate weight for many repetitions. A sample four-week beginning resistance exercise program that targets both the upper and lower body for someone in the initial stage of training is given in table 6.8.

To progress to the improvement stage, you would increase the weight you lift over the next month and then increase the repetitions. After

Table 6.8   Beginner Resistance Training Program

Monday	Tuesday	Wednesday	Thursday	Friday	Saturday	Sunday	Program change
Week 1							
Intensity: 12-14RM or 11-12 RPE Duration: 1-2 sets of 12-14 repetitions	Off or other activity	Intensity: 12-14RM or 11-12 RPE Duration: 1-2 sets of 12-14 repetitions	Off or other activity	Off or program from Mon. or Wed.	Off or other activity	Leisure or non-weight-bearing activity (gardening, swimming)	None
Week 2							
Intensity: 14-16RM or 11-12 RPE Duration: 2 sets of 14-16 repetitions	Off or other activity	Intensity: 14-16RM or 11-12 RPE Duration: 2 sets of 14-16 repetitions	Off or other activity	Off or program from Mon. or Wed.	Off or other activity	Leisure or non-weight-bearing activity (gardening, swimming)	Increased repetitions by 2-4 reps

Monday	Tuesday	Wednesday	Thursday	Friday	Saturday	Sunday	Program change
Week 3							
Intensity: 12- 14RM or 12-13 RPE *Duration:* 2 sets of 12-14 repetitions	Off or other activity	*Intensity:* 12-14RM or 12-13 RPE *Duration:* 2 sets of 12-14 repetitions	Off or other activity	Off or program from Mon. or Wed.	Off or other activity	Leisure or non-weight-bearing activity (gardening, swimming)	*Increased intensity by 2RM or 1-2 RPE*
Week 4							
Intensity: 12-14RM or 12-13 RPE *Duration:* 2-3 sets of 14-16 repetitions	Off or other activity	*Intensity:* 12-14RM or 12-13 RPE *Duration:* 2-3 sets of 14-16 repetitions	Off or other activity	Off or program from Mon. or Wed.	Off or other activity	Leisure or non-weight-bearing activity (gardening, swimming)	*Increased repetitions by 1 set and 2-4 reps*

Every exercise session would include a 5- to 10-minute warm-up before exercise and a 5- to 10-minute cool-down after exercise.

This program assumes that you would do both the lower and upper body resistance workouts in the same exercise session. Alternatively, you could perform the lower and upper body workouts on separate days (for shorter sessions) but would need to double the number of days you train.

adjusting to this level, you could increase the weight again and then the repetitions. If you wanted to add another day, you could do so later in this stage. A progression scale might look like this:

Month	Progression
2	Increase intensity by 2- to 4RM or 1 to 2 RPE (this means you will be doing two to four fewer repetitions at the higher weight).
3	Increase duration by 2 to 4 repetitions per set.
4	Increase intensity by 2- to 4RM or 1 to 2 RPE (this means you will be doing two to four fewer repetitions at the higher weight).
5	Increase duration by 2 to 4 repetitions per set.
6	Add another day per week of resistance exercise.

Intermediate Resistance Program to Improve Bone Health

If you've already been doing low- to moderate-intensity resistance exercise and want to progress to a more challenging program, you could start by increasing the weight you are lifting, then the repetitions, and then the frequency, as in the progression scale. For example, if Bob already does some light resistance exercise (13-15RM) one or two days a week but wants to move up to a more vigorous program that will help increase his bone mass, he might follow the sample program outlined in table 6.9.

Table 6.9 Intermediate Resistance Program

Monday	Tuesday	Wednesday	Thursday	Friday	Saturday	Sunday	Program change
Weeks 1-3							
Intensity: 10-12RM or 13-14 RPE *Duration:* 2-3 sets of 10-12 repetitions	Off or other activity	*Intensity:* 10-12RM or 13-14 RPE *Duration:* 2-3 sets of 10-12 repetitions	Off or other activity	*Intensity:* 10-12RM or 13-14 RPE *Duration:* 2-3 sets of 10-12 repetitions	Off or other activity	Leisure or sport activity; could be non-weight bearing	*Increased intensity of resistance exercise by 2RM or 1 RPE*
Weeks 4-6							
Intensity: 10-12RM or 13-14 RPE *Duration:* 2-3 sets of 12-14 repetitions	Off or other activity	*Intensity:* 10-12RM or 13-14 RPE *Duration:* 2-3 sets of 12-14 repetitions	Off or other activity	*Intensity:* 10- 12RM or 13-14 RPE *Duration:* 2-3 sets of 12-14 repetitions	Off or other activity	Leisure or sport activity; could be non-weight bearing	*Increased duration by 2 repetitions per set*
Weeks 7-9							
Intensity: 8-10RM or 14-15 RPE *Duration:* 2-3 sets of 8-10 repetitions	Off or other activity	*Intensity:* 8-10RM or 14-15 RPE *Duration:* 2-3 sets of 8-10 repetitions	Off or other activity	*Intensity:* 8-10RM or 14-15 RPE *Duration:* 2-3 sets of 8-10 repetitions	Off or other activity	Leisure or sport activity; could be non-weight bearing	*Increased intensity of resistance exercise by 2RM or 1 RPE*

Monday	Tuesday	Wednesday	Thursday	Friday	Saturday	Sunday	Program change
Weeks 10-12							
Intensity: 8-10RM or 14-15 RPE *Duration:* 2-3 sets of 8-10 repetitions	Off or other activity	*Intensity:* 8-10RM or 14-15 RPE *Duration:* 2-3 sets of 8-10 repetitions	Off or other activity	*Intensity:* 8-10RM or 14-15 RPE *Duration:* 2-3 sets of 8-10 repetitions	*Intensity:* 8- to 10RM or 14-15 RPE *Duration:* 2-3 sets of 8-10 repetitions	Leisure or sport activity; could be non-weight bearing	*Added another day of exercise**

Every exercise session would include a 5- to 10-minute warm-up before exercise and a 5- to 10-minute cooldown after exercise.

This program assumes that you would do both the lower and upper body resistance workouts in the same exercise session. Alternatively, you could perform the lower and upper body workouts on separate days (for shorter sessions) but would need to double the number of days you train.

After week 12 is a good time to split your program into two days each of upper and lower body exercise. If you do so, you could add a few new exercises to each workout.

To progress to the maintenance stage, Bob could slightly lower the intensity of his program and perhaps substitute an alternative activity one day per week. The first few months of a maintenance stage for the intermediate program in table 6.9 might look like this:

Maintenance stage (month)	*Program change*
1	Decrease intensity by 1- to 2RM or 1 RPE.
2	Decrease repetitions by 1 or 2 per set.
3	Substitute resistance-like activity for one day of training every other week (i.e., biking or hiking on a course with hills, kayaking, or rowing).

Adding Impact Exercise

Impact exercise such as jumping can improve or maintain bone mass of the hip and can help strengthen the legs. Impact exercise would be most suited for people who have osteopenia of the hip and want to improve their bone mass and for those with mild osteoporosis of the hip who have received physician clearance to begin such a program. Impact exercise is not suitable for women with moderate to advanced osteoporosis or those who have had a recent fracture. If you are significantly overweight or have a history of joint problems, other types of exercise may be more appropriate for you.

To challenge the skeleton, the impact must be of moderate to vigorous intensity. Several types of sport exercise have periods of impact activity and can promote bone health. Examples of impact sports are volleyball, basketball, gymnastics, and wrestling. High-impact aerobic dance and running are other types of exercise that include an impact component. Simple jumping exercise, such as jumping in place or hopping on one foot, is a quick and simple activity to add to your existing exercise program to get bone benefits. Sample jumping programs are described later in the chapter, and sample exercises and illustrations of proper jumping technique are given in chapter 7.

Gauging Intensity

The intensity of impact exercise is harder to gauge than it is for aerobic and resistance training. The only way to truly measure impact intensity is with laboratory instruments. However, we do know from simple laws of physics that jumping intensity can be increased by jumping higher or jumping with added weight. Progressing to higher intensity jumping, such as jumping onto and off of an exercise step or with a weighted vest (see chapter 7), should be reserved for people who do not have osteoporosis and who have a base of lower body strength (see "Building a Base for Jumping"). Simple jumping exercises are fine for most people without advanced osteoporosis or joint limitations.

Building a Base for Jumping

Because of the stress impact exercise places on the joints, it is important for them to be surrounded by strong muscles and connective tissues to avoid injury. In our programs, we have found that for beginning jumpers, doing two to three months of lower body resistance exercise prior to adding jumping helps prepare the muscles and joints for impact training and greatly reduces the risk of injury. If you do not participate in any impact activities and want to add jumping to your program, it would be best to add a few lower body resistance exercises for a couple of months before starting to jump. If you are already active in activities that have built a base of leg strength, it is probably safe for you to begin a moderate-intensity jumping program.

Beginner Jump Training Program for Hip Bone Health

If you have mild osteoporosis or do not currently do any impact exercise, you should start at the beginning level. For two to three months *prior* to this, you should follow the beginning exercise program for lower body resistance exercise described previously. After you've built up some leg strength, you can add jumping. Table 6.10 gives a sample four-week beginning jumping program for someone in the initial stage of training.

Table 6.10 Beginner Jump Training Program

Monday	Tuesday	Wednesday	Thursday	Friday	Saturday	Sunday	Program change
Week 1							
3 sets of 6 jumps		3 sets of 6 jumps		3 sets of 6 jumps			None
Week 2							
4 sets of 8 jumps		4 sets of 8 jumps		4 sets of 8 jumps			Increased by 1 set and 2 reps
Week 3							
4 sets of 8 jumps		4 sets of 10 jumps		4 sets of 10 jumps			Increased by 2 reps
Week 4							
5 sets of 10 jumps		5 sets of 10 jumps		5 sets of 10 jumps			Increased by 1 set

Jumps are easily added to the end of any aerobic, resistance, or stretching program.

Jumps should not be done without some form of warm-up, but since the workout is short, it may not require a cool-down period if done alone.

To progress to the improvement stage, you could increase the total number of jumps performed by increasing the sets and repetitions of jumping or adding another day of jump training. A progression scale might look like this:

Month	*Progression*
2	Increase jumps to 12 repetitions per set.
3	Add one or two sets of jumps.
4	Add an additional day of jumping.

If you have osteoporosis or other limitations, you should then progress to a maintenance stage by sticking to your jump training routine. For variety, you could substitute a fun impact activity such as aerobic dance class once or twice a week.

Intermediate Jump Training Program for Hip Bone Health

After you've been jumping for some time and have a base of lower body strength, you may wish to progress to a more rigorous program. You could increase the jump intensity by increasing the height of or adding weight to your jumps. To increase the height of jumps, you can jump onto and off of a step bench, such as that used in aerobic dance classes. To increase the force of a jump, you can wear a weighted vest that makes the bone challenge produced by jumping even greater. A sample program for jumping exercise in the intermediate stage is outlined in table 6.11.

Table 6.11 Intermediate Jump Training Program

Monday	Tuesday	Wednesday	Thursday	Friday	Saturday	Sunday	Program change
Weeks 1-3							
Intensity: jump onto 4-in. step* *Duration:* 5 sets of 10 jumps	Off or other activity	*Intensity:* jump onto 4-in. step *Duration:* 5 sets of 10 jumps	Off or other activity	*Intensity:* jump onto 4-in. step *Duration:* 5 sets of 10 jumps	Off or other activity	Leisure or sport activity	*Increased jump intensity by adding 4-in. step*
Weeks 4-6							
Intensity: jump onto 4-in. step *Duration:* 6 sets of 10 jumps	Off or other activity	*Intensity:* jump onto 4-in. step *Duration:* 6 sets of 10 jumps	Off or other activity	*Intensity:* jump onto 4-in. step *Duration:* 7 sets of 10 jumps	Off or other activity	Leisure or sport activity	*Increased by 1-2 sets*
Weeks 7-9							
Intensity: jump onto 8-in. step *Duration:* 6 sets of 10 jumps	Off or other activity	*Intensity:* jump onto 8-in. step *Duration:* 7 sets of 10 jumps	Off or other activity	*Intensity:* jump onto 8-in. step *Duration:* 7 sets of 10 jumps	Off or other activity	Leisure or sport activity	*Added second 4-in. step*
Weeks 10-12							
Intensity: jump onto 8-in. step *Duration:* 5-7 sets of 10 jumps	Off or other activity	*Intensity:* jump onto 8-in. step *Duration:* 5-7 sets of 10 jumps	Off or other activity	*Intensity:* jump onto 8-in. step *Duration:* 5-7 sets of 10 jumps	*Intensity:* jump onto 8-in. step *Duration:* 7 sets of 10 jumps	Leisure or sport activity	*Added another day of jumping*

*Exercise step bench is 4 inches high and can be acquired commercially, but is usually standard equipment in gyms and health clubs; alternatively, you could jump onto and off of some other stable surface.

Jumps are easily added to the end of any aerobic, resistance, or stretching program.

Jumps should not be done without some form of warm-up, but since the workout is short, it may not require a cool-down period if done alone.

Adding Balance Exercise

Maintaining balance while standing or moving in your environment is key in preventing falls. Although strengthening your leg muscles will contribute to better balance, certain exercises can specifically challenge the other systems that help maintain your stability. However, fall prevention research has shown that balance exercises alone are not enough to prevent falls, but when combined with resistance training, they become an effective strategy for fall prevention. Balance exercises are suitable for most people as long as proper technique and safety guidelines are followed. Balance exercises may be especially important for people who have osteoporosis, have a history of falls, or have experienced a fracture.

The intensity of balance exercises cannot be measured in the same way that aerobic and resistance exercise can, but some exercises may be more challenging to perform than others. Most balance exercises require you to hold a position for a certain length of time or to do several repetitions of a particular movement. To challenge your balance systems, exercises should be difficult yet not impossible to perform. To progress, you can increase the length of time you hold a position, increase repetitions of a particular movement, or add more difficult moves. Since balance exercises do not require physical recovery, you can perform them every day. Some of my research participants tell me that they practice standing on one leg whenever they are waiting in line at the grocery store or post office. You may get some awkward stares, but this is a perfect way to incorporate some exercise into your daily routine! Examples of effective balance exercises are described and illustrated in chapter 7.

Combined Exercise Programs

Depending on your goals, you may wish to combine several types of activity to best optimize your overall health. Osteoporosis is likely not your only health concern, and you may have other chronic illnesses that you need to manage. Since the principle of specificity tells us that different types of exercise may be most useful for particular health goals, you may think you have to do a lot of exercise to target your total health. But you can accomplish this without being overwhelmed by being a good manager of your exercise time. You can do different types of exercises on different days of the week or you can do shorter bouts of different types of exercise in one multi-exercise session. Tables 6.12 and 6.13 provide examples of each method of combining your exercise programs.

Fall-Prevention Program

If the goal of your exercise program is to prevent falls, you should focus on a program of walking combined with lower body resistance exercise and balance exercise (Kohrt et al. 2004). Walking will help improve your

Table 6.12 Combined Aerobic and Resistance Exercise Program Varied by Day

Monday	Tuesday	Wednesday	Thursday	Friday	Saturday	Sunday
30-45 min aerobic	30-45 min resistance	30-45 min aerobic	Off or alternative activity (i.e., yoga, hiking)	30-45 min resistance	30-45 min aerobic	Off or alternative activity (i.e., stretching, tai chi)
Stretching	Stretching	Stretching	Stretching	Stretching	Stretching	Stretching

Table 6.13 Combined Aerobic and Resistance Exercise Program Varied Within a Session

Monday	Tuesday	Wednesday	Thursday	Friday	Saturday	Sunday
20-30 min aerobic 15-20 min LB resistance	Off or alternative activity (i.e., stretching, hiking)	20-30 min aerobic 15-20 min UB resistance	20-30 min aerobic 15-20 min LB resistance	Off or alternative activity (i.e., yoga, tai chi)	20-30 min aerobic 15-20 min UB resistance	Off or alternative activity (i.e., yoga, hiking)
Stretching	Stretching	Stretching	Stretching	Stretching	Stretching	Stretching

LB = lower body

UB = upper body

mobility and gait by challenging the muscles and systems responsible for keeping you steady while moving. Lower body resistance exercise will help strengthen muscles used for balance during standing and while in motion and will improve your ability to recover from a slip, trip, or stumble. Specific balance exercise can help lower fall risk by challenging the nerves and muscles that keep you steady. Table 6.14 presents a sample fall-prevention exercise program.

Alternative Forms of Exercise

Forms of exercise that are indigenous to other parts of the world may offer alternatives for supplementing a standard training program such as those described here. Tai chi and yoga are two forms of exercise that contain elements which may help prevent falls. Both have their origins in Asia and have been used to promote physical and mental well-being.

Table 6.14 Fall-Prevention Program

Monday	Tuesday	Wednesday	Thursday	Friday	Saturday	Sunday
15-20 min walk 15 min LB resistance 5 min balance 5-10 min stretching	Balance Flexibility	15-20 min walk 15 min LB resistance 5 min balance 5-10 min stretching	15-20 min walk 15 min LB resistance 5 min balance 5-10 min stretching	5 min balance 5-10 min stretching	Recreational physical activity (e.g., hiking or gardening)	Off or alternative activity

LB = lower body

Tai chi emphasizes slow, coordinated movements throughout the range of motion, often while moving the body away from its center of mass so as to challenge dynamic balance. Research studies have shown that tai chi exercise effectively reduces falls among older adults. In one study, tai chi prevented falls better than a balance training program that used computerized balance equipment (Wolf et al.1996). Although the exact reasons why tai chi prevents falls are still being studied, some hypothesize that it improves leg strength, mobility, and balance—all key risk factors for falls.

Yoga is an ancient form of exercise that usually involves holding several different postures for a period of time and also emphasizes controlled breathing. Although yoga is not specifically studied for preventing falls, it can promote strength and balance, which are important elements of a fall-prevention program.

Tai chi and yoga are often taught in a class format at private facilities, health clubs, or community centers, and home videos for both types of exercise programs are also available commercially. If you decide to add an alternative form of exercise such as tai chi or yoga to your regular exercise program, be sure to choose a class or tape that is appropriate for your initial fitness level and that is not too easy or too hard. The best way to assess this is to talk with the class instructor or, for videos, to read the detailed information on the video or look for a review of it on the Internet. Most Internet video sale sites have customer reviews and ratings of their products.

Summary

In this chapter, we've gotten to the heart of what is needed to begin an exercise program aimed at improving your bone health. If you are a beginning exerciser or are already exercising and want to progress to the next level, fill out the PAR-Q to assess whether you need to seek the advice of a physician before beginning your new exercise program. If you have never exercised before, you should discuss your plans to start exercising with your doctor and consider starting off with a simple walking program that will get you used to exercise and ready to move to the next level. Setting realistic and achievable goals will help you determine the type of program that will improve your overall health and motivate you to keep exercising. I've provided several sample exercise programs based on various types of activity and starting fitness levels. You don't have to follow these sample programs, but they may give you an idea of how to plan your exercise program so that it is most effective at improving your bone health.

ACTION PLAN:
CREATING A CUSTOMIZED EXERCISE PLAN

- ☐ Fill out the PAR-Q to determine whether you are ready to exercise. If not, consult your physician about beginning an exercise program.
- ☐ Set both short- and long-term goals for your exercise program.
- ☐ Review the sample exercise programs described in this chapter and follow or modify the program best suited to your abilities, preferences, and goals.
- ☐ Understand how to determine the intensity of your aerobic or resistance program.
- ☐ Consider supplementing your regular exercise program with an alternative form of exercise such as tai chi or yoga.

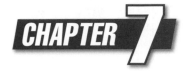

BENEFITING FROM PROPER TECHNIQUE

In this chapter, I describe suggested exercises, techniques, and tips for the programs discussed in chapter 6. Where possible, I've included a photograph that shows proper form and execution for selected exercises. When starting out, you will benefit by exercising with a partner who can give you feedback about your execution and form. Health club trainers can also help you with your technique. If you don't have a partner to exercise with or a professional to advise you, you could begin by exercising in a room with a full-length mirror so you can evaluate your own form and technique. Walls in health clubs are mirrored for that exact reason. Most of us don't like to watch ourselves exercise, but you should do so from time to time so you can check for proper technique, which in turn ensures the most effective and safe workout. If you exercise alone without a mirror, you need to pay special attention to your body for signs of unusual joint or muscle pain. Many exercise-related injuries are due to poor form that is easily corrected. If you begin to notice such pain, you should find a way to evaluate your form or consult with a professional for guidance.

Some people think that exercise can only be performed in a health club and are immediately turned off by the proposition. Others prefer to exercise at health clubs because they offer a variety of programs, specialized equipment, and professional instruction. The truth is that you can exercise virtually *anyplace* and often with minimal equipment. In this chapter, where appropriate, I provide descriptions for doing exercises in both the home and health club settings. Chapter 10 includes more information on deciding where to exercise and what equipment you'll need. The most important factor in choosing an exercise setting is finding one that will help you reach your goals and maintain a lifelong plan.

Aerobic Exercise

Aerobic exercise can be done at home or at a gym, with minimal to more extensive equipment, alone or in a class, indoors or outdoors. The beauty of aerobic exercise is that there are many options, so it is easy to find activities that are effective and that suit your preferences and needs. Remember that bone-building and bone-maintaining exercise should be weight bearing and should be a little more vigorous than walking. Table 6.2 on page 71 lists several examples of aerobic exercise types that have effectively improved bone health in women, and chapter 6 includes sample beginning and intermediate programs.

Form is important for aerobic exercise because poor form can place unusual stresses and strains on your body, which over time could lead to injury. For most weight-bearing exercises, this means you should maintain a stable upright posture with your core muscles (back, abdomen, pelvis) in alignment at all times. For lower body exercise (e.g., jogging or stepping), your arms and shoulders should be relaxed. Figure 7.1 shows proper form for aerobic exercise. If you exercise on aerobic equipment, make sure you get proper instruction or study the manual for information on proper form and use of the equipment. When in doubt, consult with a professional. Figures 7.2 and 7.3 show examples of proper form on

Proper Aerobic Exercise Technique

Aerobic exercise usually increases your body temperature, so you will feel different 10 to 15 minutes into your program compared to when you started. Ensure adequate ventilation, particularly when exercising indoors.

- ▸ Dress appropriately.
- ▸ Wear breathable fabrics.
- ▸ Dress in layers in cold weather so you can remove layers if you get too warm.
- ▸ Wear a hat in warm or cold weather.

Wear UV protection in sunny weather or higher altitudes (sunscreen, sunglasses, hat).

Maintain proper form.

Self-monitor intensity regularly. Slow down if you are exercising too hard.

Stop exercising if you experience unusual shortness of breath or pain.

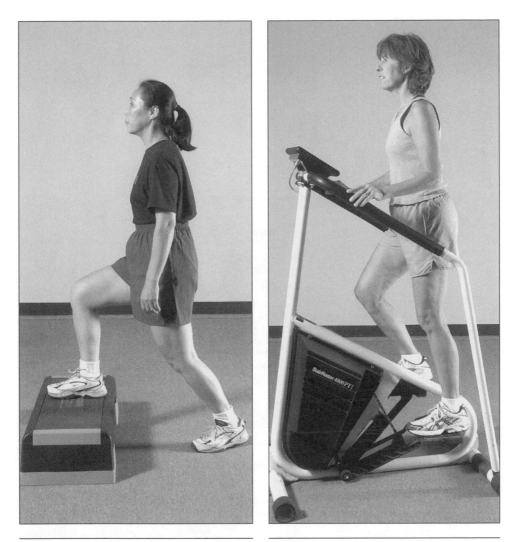

Figure 7.1 Proper form during bench step aerobic exercise.

Figure 7.2 Proper form on a stair climber.

the stair climber and rowing machine. Make sure the equipment has an emergency stop button. For the safety of pets or small children, do not exercise when they are present.

Resistance Exercise

Resistance exercise can also be done at home or at a gym but usually requires at least minimal equipment and is often, but not always, performed individually. A wide variety of equipment is available for resistance training. Sample beginning and intermediate programs are described in chapter 6.

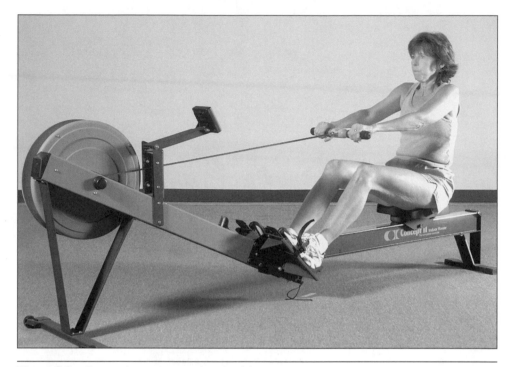

Figure 7.3   Proper form on a rowing machine.

Equipment

Equipment is usually categorized as machine or free weight, but new equipment is being developed all the time. Each type of equipment has advantages and limitations.

Resistance machines are most common in gym settings but can also be purchased for home use. Machines allow you to work isolated muscle groups, such as the biceps or triceps, and help the beginning exerciser maintain proper form. However, machines are costly (in terms of either gym fees or purchase price), and fewer exercises can be done in a weight-bearing position, an important factor when exercising for bone and functional health.

Free weights typically include a barbell with plates of varying weight and one or more sets of handheld dumbbells of varying weight. These two types of equipment allow you to apply resistance to both upper and lower body movements. Advantages of free weights are a low equipment cost and the additional strengthening of accessory muscles used to stabilize your body when performing a movement. For example, when you are standing for a biceps curl using a barbell, not only are you working your biceps, but you are working your legs and back to stabilize yourself as you execute the lift. Maintaining form during free-weight exercise is challenging, so exercising with the correct weights is important. When in doubt, err on the conservative side with a lighter weight. If you are investing in free weights for home use, try out the weights in the store to make sure you have the correct amount. In my case, one barbell with adjustable weights and a set of 12- and 20-pound dumbbells allow me to do most exercises within my target range. The barbell is used for the heaviest weight, about 40 pounds, that I use to exercise large muscle groups such as my legs, back, and chest. The 20-pound dumbbells are used to exercise my stronger small muscle groups (e.g., isolated back areas and biceps and triceps), whereas the 12-pound dumbbells are used to exercise my smallest and weakest muscle groups (e.g., shoulders). Limitations of using free weights include a challenge to maintain form, the need for workout space and storage space, and modest financial cost.

Other resistance equipment includes elastic bands or tubing, exercise balls, and weighted vests. Most can be found in sporting goods stores or on the Internet. Elastic bands and tubing are similar to free weights and allow you to do many types of exercise by pulling or moving against the resistance of the band or tubing. Imagine a very large, thick rubber band and think about how much strength you'd have to use to stretch it. Or imagine someone with a bow and arrow who has to use muscle force to pull back the arrow against the elastic resistance of the bowstring. Elastic bands and tubing come in a variety of resistances that reflect how stretchy or stiff the elastic is. Often the different intensities are color coded so that you can easily distinguish resistance levels. You can adjust your grip on the bands to change the tautness. Bringing your hands closer together on the band makes the exercise more challenging, and spacing your hands further apart makes the exercise a little easier. If you have trouble gripping the ends of the band because of arthritis or weakness, you can use special handles and other gripping aids that are sold as accessories to the bands. Advantages of using elastic resistance are low expense and portability of the equipment. Limitations include an adjustment period for getting used to the proper form and technique when using bands and a potential upper limit to the intensity that can be achieved without sacrificing form.

Exercise balls are common equipment these days. These oversized rubber balls can be used for therapeutic purposes and for some resistance exercises. I even sit on one in my office because it reduces the pressure on my back. Exercise balls are fun and effective, but for the sake of space, I do not present examples of exercise using balls. If you are interested in exploring this option, I recommend you look for published exercise guides and videos for ball exercise. Exercise balls do present some risk of falling, so you need to follow instructions carefully and use common sense.

Weighted vests are gaining in popularity as a training tool. Although they are not standard equipment in gyms or sporting goods stores, they are available through the Internet or specialty stores. Exercising with a weighted vest is analogous to exercising while wearing a backpack. A weighted vest is usually made of some type of breathable and durable fabric and contains many small sleeves that hold small, rod-shaped weights, usually weighing one or two pounds each. You can fill the vest with weights in small increments to progress your training gradually and safely. Weighted vests are worn during lower body exercise to provide resistance. They are safer than barbells because the weight is carried close to your body and distributed evenly so that you are not put off balance and do not incur awkward strains. We have used weighted vests in many of our exercise studies in populations from 13 to 90 years of age. Our participants like exercising with vests because they do not have to hold anything and are more stable and because they can adjust the weight in small increments. I do not recommend making your own version of a weighted vest with a backpack or fishing vest (this has been attempted!) because the weight is difficult to distribute evenly and can thus be unsafe. Weighted vests offer several advantages, including safety, portability, and the ability to adjust weight in small increments. Disadvantages include a small financial investment (average cost is $100) and their limited application for lower body resistance only.

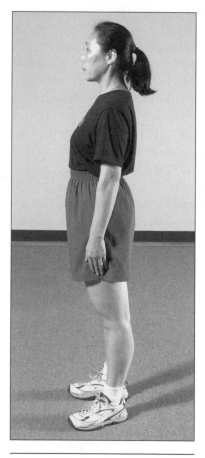

Figure 7.4 In a stable upright posture, the core muscles (back, abdomen, and pelvis) are in alignment and the neck is in a neutral position.

Proper Form

Doing a resistance exercise with proper form is critically important because poor form reduces the effectiveness of exercise and often leads to injury. For exercises done in a standing position, you should maintain a stable upright posture with your core muscles (back, abdomen, pelvis) in alignment at all times (see figure 7.4). For seated exercise, also make sure that you are in proper position at the start and during the movement. It is easy to slip into poor form on equipment when you are tired, so if you find yourself doing so, you may need to lower the intensity of your workout or stop altogether. Descriptions and illustrations of proper form for selected exercises are provided in the following sections. The sidebar on page 115 offers tips on proper resistance exercise technique.

Resistance Exercise Descriptions

Following are some resistance exercises for the upper and lower body—options for you to incorporate into your resistance training program. Before performing an exercise, read the description carefully and be guided by the photos to ensure proper technique and avoid injury.

CHEST PRESS

Works the chest and arms

Starting position: In standing position, wrap an exercise band or tubing around your back and grip one end with each hand, about 6 to 12 inches from the end. The starting position for this exercise is with your arms bent and your hands beside your chest, slightly in front of and just under your armpits.

Movement: Push your hands forward, extending your arms straight out. Do this for a count of three seconds and, after a full extension, bring the band or tubing back to the starting position for another count of three. You should feel your chest and arms working. You may need to alter your grip on the band or tubing slightly forward if the movement was too hard or slightly back if the movement was too easy.

Free-weight version: To do this exercise with free weights, you will need some type of bench to lie on. Holding a dumbbell in each hand, you use the same starting position and movement as for the band or tubing version except that you are lying flat on your back instead of standing up.

Machine version: The bench press is similar to a chest press and is done in a supine (flat on your back) position. Some weight machines also allow you to do a chest press in a seated position.

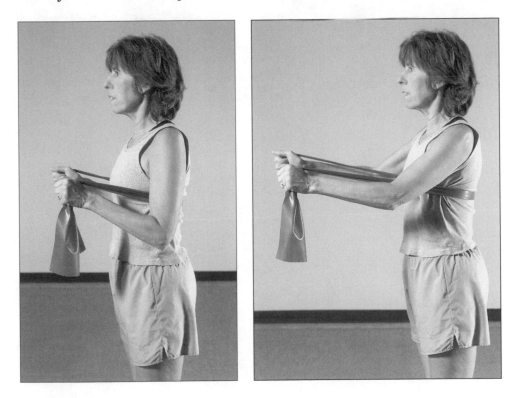

CHEST FLY

Works the chest and arms

Starting position: In standing position, wrap an exercise band or tubing around your upper back and grip the band or tubing near the ends. The starting position for this exercise is with your arms outstretched and to your sides at shoulder level and parallel to the ground.

Movement: Keeping your arms straight, bring your hands together so that they are straight out in front of you. Do this for a count of three seconds, and after your hands touch slightly, bring the band or tubing back to the starting position for another count of three. You may need to alter your grip on the band or tubing slightly forward if the movement was too hard or slightly back if the movement was too easy.

Free-weight version: To do this exercise with free weights, you will need some type of bench to lie on. Holding a dumbbell in each hand, you use the same starting position and movement as for the band or tubing version except that you are lying flat on your back instead of standing up.

Machine version: Some weight machines allow you to do a chest fly in a seated position.

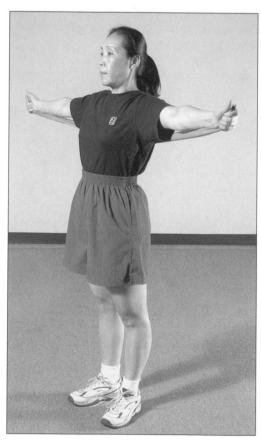 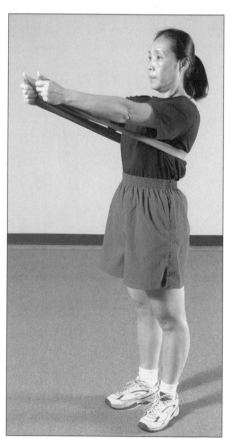

ARM PULL-DOWN

Works the back and shoulders

Starting position: Begin in a standing position and grasp the band or tubing with both hands near the middle and both arms extended overhead.

Movement: Pull the band or tubing downward with both arms at the same time, keeping your arms straight and ending with your arms outstretched to each side. Do this for a count of three seconds until your arms are at shoulder level and then bring the band or tubing back to the starting position for another count of three. You should feel your shoulders and back working. You may need to alter your grip on the band or tubing slightly toward the ends if the movement was too hard or slightly away from the ends if the movement was too easy.

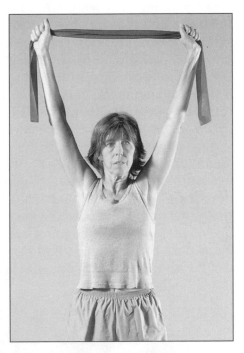

Horizontal version: For this version, you start with your arms directly in front of you at shoulder height instead of overhead. The movement is similar to the previous version except that you pull the band or tubing backward until your arms are fully extended out to each side.

Machine version: There is a seated version of this exercise, which can also be called the "latissimus dorsi pull-down" or "lat pull-down."

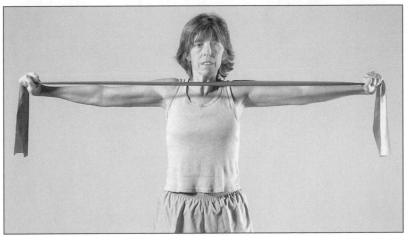

ONE-ARM ROW (OR BOW AND ARROW)

Works the back and arms

Starting position: In standing position with both arms in front of you at shoulder level, grasp near the middle of the band or tubing with both hands. Bend your left arm and place your left hand just in front of your right shoulder. Keep your right arm extended out to your right side, parallel to the ground.

Movement: Pull your left hand across your chest, keeping your elbow bent, so that your left hand ends up in front of your left shoulder and just slightly under your armpit (as in pulling an arrow back from the bow). Do this for a count of three seconds until your arm is all the way over, then bring the band or tubing back to the starting position for another count of three. You should feel your arm and the right side of your back working. You may need to alter your grip on the band or tubing slightly back if the movement was too hard or slightly forward if the movement was too easy. After you've finished all of your reps on the left side, switch so that you are working the right side of your back.

Free-weight version: To do this exercise with free weights, you will need some type of bench to prop yourself. Start by putting your left knee and left hand on the bench so that your back is parallel to the bench. With a dumbbell in your right hand, start by keeping your arm fully extended so that your right hand is below the level of the bench. Then pull the weight up in a straight line, bending your elbow and finishing with your right hand next to your chest and just under your armpit. Slowly lower the weight and repeat with the left side after you've completed your repetitions for the right.

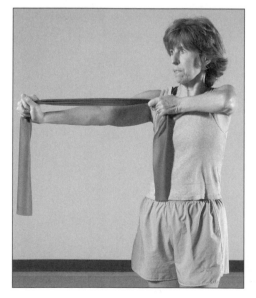 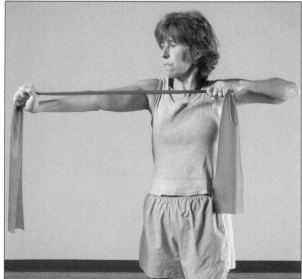

SEATED ROW

Works the back and arms

Starting position: Begin by sitting on the floor with your legs extended in front of you, with your knees slightly bent and your feet flexed. Wrap the band or tubing around your feet and grasp it with both hands, keeping your arms fully extended (where you grasp depends on the length of the band or tubing and your strength). Your back should be straight and tilted just slightly forward. *You should not bend your back and drop your head forward.*

Movement: Pulling with both arms at the same time, bring the band or tubing toward you by bending your elbows and drawing your hands next to your sides. Do this for a count of three seconds, and after your arms are fully back, bring the band or tubing back to the starting position for another count of three. You should feel your arms and back working.

Your back should not move, but should stay in the starting position throughout the movement while only your hands move. You may need to alter your grip on the band or tubing slightly toward the ends if the movement was too hard or slightly away from the ends if the movement was too easy.

Machine version: There is a machine version of the seated row. Some machines have you sit on the floor and others have you sit on a seat with your chest stabilized against a cushioned bar. The starting positions and movements are nearly the same as for the band or tubing version.

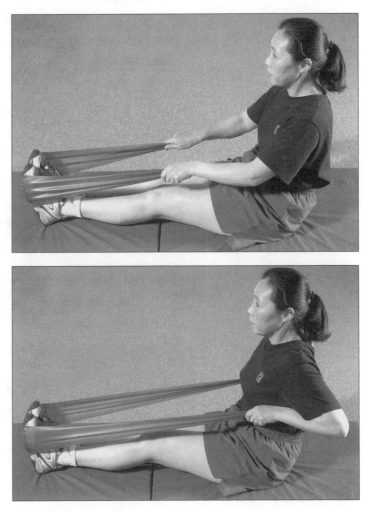

UPRIGHT ROW

Works the back and arms

Starting position: Begin in a standing position with one foot slightly in front of the other and step on the band or tubing with the front foot. Grasp the band or tubing near the ends, with your right arm extended and your hand just in front of your lead leg.

Movement: Pull the band or tubing upward by bending your elbow out and raising your hand until it is just in front of your chest and beneath your chin. Do this for a count of three seconds, and when your hand is just under your chin, bring the band or tubing back to the starting position for another count of three. You should feel your shoulders and back working. You may need to alter your grip on the band or tubing slightly toward the ends if the movement was too hard or slightly away from the ends

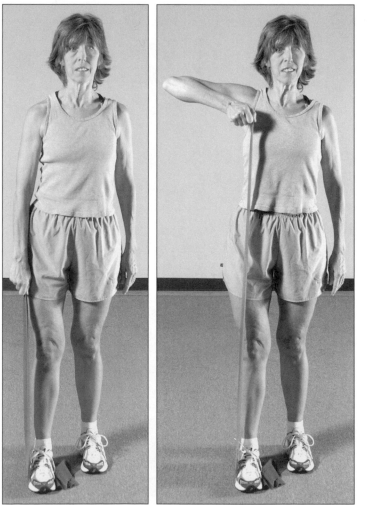

if the movement was too easy. Remember to switch arms and work the other side.

Free-weight version: In a standing position, grasp a barbell with both hands so that it rests just in front of the top of your thigh. The movement is the same as for the band or tubing version except that you pull up with both arms simultaneously.

SIDE SHOULDER RAISE

Works the back and middle part of the shoulders

Starting position: Begin in a standing position and step on the band or tubing with your right foot. Grasp the band or tubing near the end with your right hand and arm extended and resting beside your right hip.

Movement: Keeping your arm straight, raise your hand until it is at the same level as your shoulder or slightly above. Do this for a count of three seconds, and after your arm is raised, bring the band or tubing back to the starting position for another count of three. You should feel your shoulders working. You may need to alter your grip on the band or tubing slightly toward the ends if the movement was too hard or slightly away from the ends if the movement was too easy. After you've completed all repetitions with your right hand, switch to your left hand and complete your set.

Free-weight version: In a standing position, grasp a dumbbell with your right hand so that it rests to the right of the top of your thigh. The movement is the same as for the band or tubing version. Remember to exercise both arms.

Machine version: There is a seated machine version of this exercise, but in that version you are usually raising both arms simultaneously.

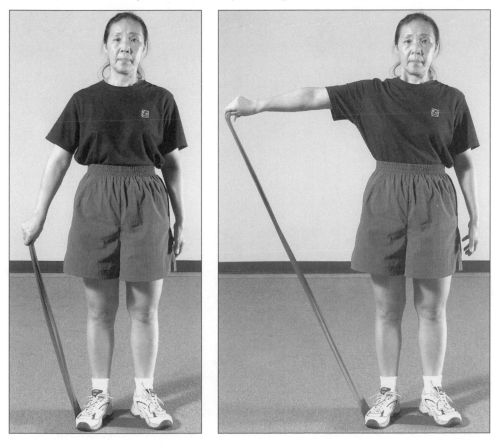

FRONT SHOULDER RAISE

Works the back and front part of the shoulders

Starting position: Begin in a standing position and step on the band or tubing with your right foot. Grasp the band or tubing near the end with your right hand and arm extended and resting near the front of your right thigh.

Movement: Keeping your arm straight, raise your hand until it is at the same level as your shoulder or slightly above. Do this for a count of three seconds, and after your arm is raised, bring the band or tubing back to the starting position for another count of three. You should feel your shoulders working. You may need to alter your grip on the band or tubing slightly toward the ends if the movement was too hard or slightly away from the ends if the movement was too easy. After you've completed all repetitions with your right hand, switch to your left and complete your set.

Free-weight version: In a standing position, grasp a dumbbell with your right hand so that it rests on top of your thigh. The movement is the same as for the band or tubing version. Remember to exercise both arms.

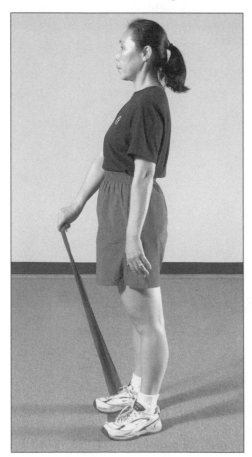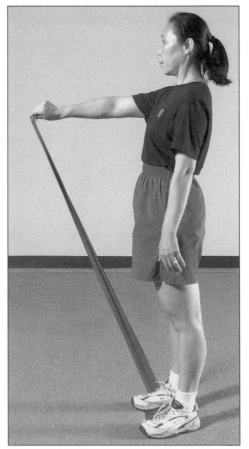

BICEPS CURL (SINGLE- OR DOUBLE-ARM)

Works the front of the arms

Starting position: Begin in a standing position with the right foot a step in front of the left and your knees slightly bent. Wrap the band or tubing underneath your right leg, just under the knee joint, and grasp the band or tubing on each side. Keep your arms extended downward and stabilize your upper arms against your sides.

Movement: Pulling with both arms at the same time, raise the band or tubing upward by bending your elbows. The movement is complete when your palms are directly facing the front of your shoulders. Do this for a count of three seconds, and after your arms are fully flexed, bring the band or tubing back to the starting position for another count of three. You should feel the front of your arms working. You may need to alter your grip on the band or tubing slightly toward the ends if the movement was too hard or slightly away from the ends if the movement was too easy. *Note:* During this movement, keep your upper arms steady and along your sides. Keep your back straight, and avoid using your back as you bring your arms up. If you find you cannot complete the exercise without swinging your upper arms or back forward, you probably had too much

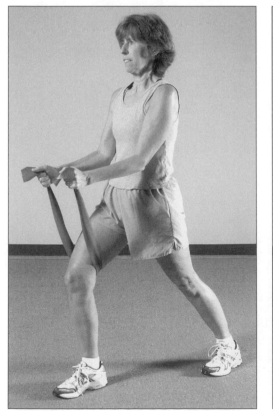 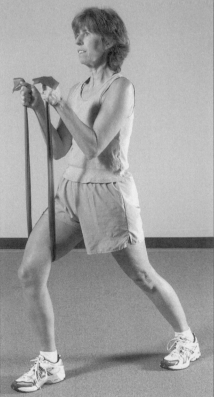

tension on the band at the start and need to readjust your hand position; if you are already at the end of the band or tubing, you'll need to use one with lower tension.

One-arm version: The starting position for this version is the same as for the shoulder raise. The movement is the same as that described for the double-arm curl except that you are only using one arm. Since this version is more difficult, you may have to reduce the starting tension on the band.

Free-weight version: You could do the biceps curl exercise in a standing position using a barbell. You would grip the barbell with your hands about shoulder-width apart. You could also do a one-arm biceps curl with a dumbbell, but these are usually done in a seated position to reduce the tendency to use your back during the movement.

Machine version: There is a seated version of the double-arm biceps curl, which can also be called a "preacher curl."

TRICEPS EXTENSION

Works the back of the arms

Starting position: The starting position is the same as for the one-arm row (bow and arrow) except that each hand is directly in front of the same shoulder. The elbows are bent out to the sides and at shoulder level.

Movement: Extend your right arm completely by moving your right hand in an arc in front of you and ending with your arm completely outstretched to your right side. Do this for a count of three seconds, and after your arm is fully extended, bring the band or tubing back to the starting position for another count of three. You should feel the back of your arms working. You may need to alter your grip on the band or tubing outward if the movement was too hard or slightly inward if the movement was too easy. After you've completed all reps for the right side, switch to the left side and complete your set.

Free-weight version: This version is similar to the band or tubing version except you raise your arm directly overhead instead of to the side. Begin by holding a dumbbell with your right hand, your arm fully bent and your elbow pointing straight up in the air. The dumbbell should be slightly touching the back of your right shoulder. Use your left hand to keep your upper right arm steady as you extend your right arm and lift the weight directly overhead. Don't forget to exercise both arms.

Machine version: There is a seated machine version of the triceps extension. Another machine version is done with both arms extending simultaneously.

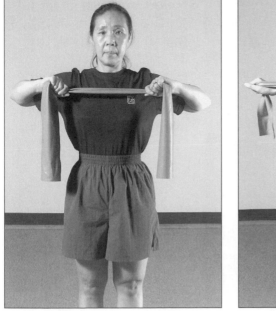 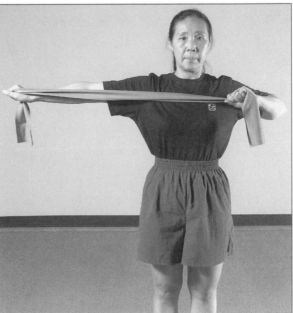

TRICEPS DIP

Works the back of the arms

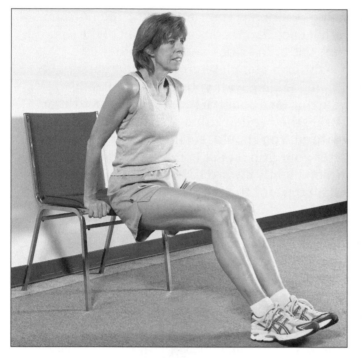

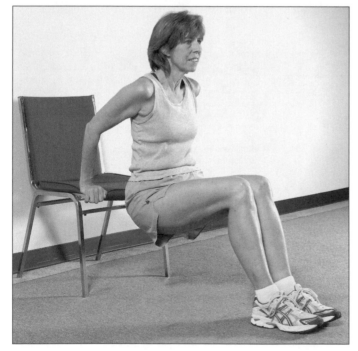

Starting position: Place a steady chair (i.e., without wheels or casters) against a wall with the seat facing out. From a seated position, place your hands palm down on the edge of the chair on each side of you. Slowly raise your buttocks off the seat and just in front of the chair edge. Walk your feet out in front of you until your legs are partially extended.

Movement: Keeping all parts of your body still, lower your body in front of the chair by bending your arms at the elbows, then push yourself back up by straightening your arms. Start by lowering just slightly on the first repetition, then try to increase the amount on succeeding repetitions. The farther you lower yourself, the more challenging it will be to push yourself back up.

SQUAT

Works the thighs and buttocks

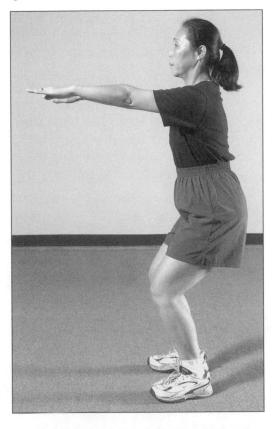

Starting position: Stand with your back straight and your feet a little wider than shoulder-width apart. If you are a beginning exerciser, you can start with a wider stance and turn your toes outward (this takes some pressure off your knees).

Movement: Slowly lower your buttocks toward the floor, as if you were going to sit down in a chair, until your legs are bent between 45 and 90 degrees. (How far down you go will depend on your strength. Start at 45 degrees, and as you get stronger, try to go lower. It is very hard to get to 90 degrees.) Slowly return to the starting position. *Note:* Try to keep your back as straight as possible, and resist bending forward at the waist. Your knees should be just over your toes (not past them!) at all times. This will be difficult, and you can make it easier by remembering to keep your buttocks back and your heels on the floor. It may also help to keep your arms out in front of you for counterbalance. If this exercise is too difficult for you to do without losing balance, start with the chair raise until you have built up more strength.

Free-weight version: You can do this exercise and many other lower body exercises with a dumbbell in each hand. Free weights are more challenging for maintaining balance, so you should have experience doing these movements and begin with very light weight. A weighted vest is a perfect way to make this exercise more challenging.

Band or tubing version: You can do this exercise with a band. Step on the band with both feet and grip the ends of the band with your hands, keeping your arms at shoulder level. Follow the same movement as for the regular squat.

Machine version: See the leg press.

CHAIR RAISE

Works the thighs and buttocks

Starting position: Sit at the edge of a stable, straight-backed chair with your back straight and your feet a little wider than shoulder-width apart and directly under your knees (your lower and upper leg should be at a right angle). Cross your arms across your chest (helps you avoid using your arms).

Movement: Slowly raise yourself out of the chair to a full stand. Concentrate on using your legs to lift yourself. Slowly return to the starting position. Do not just plop back into the chair, as you will be working muscles on your way down as well!

Band or tubing version: See the squat.

Machine version: See the leg press.

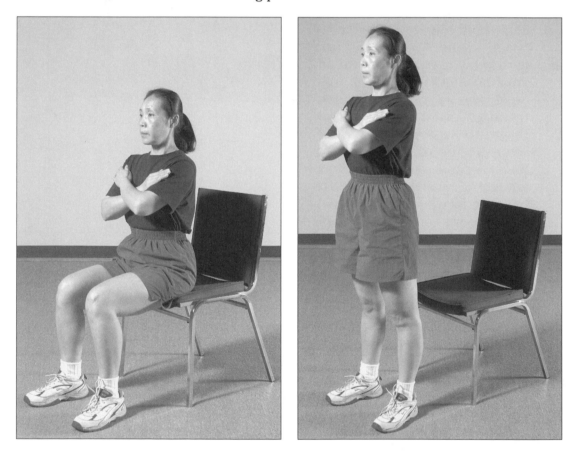

LEG PRESS

Works the thighs and buttocks

Starting position: You will usually begin this exercise in a seated (shown here) or slightly reclined position. Adjust the seat so that both your torso and upper legs and your upper and lower legs are at right angles. Cross you arms across your chest. *Note:* I suggest not using the handles provided under most seats as there is a tendency to use them to incorporate your back muscles into the movement.

Movement: Slowly extend your legs until there is just a slight bend in your knees. *Do not completely extend your legs or lock your knees.* Slowly return to the starting position.

Band or tubing version: See the squat.

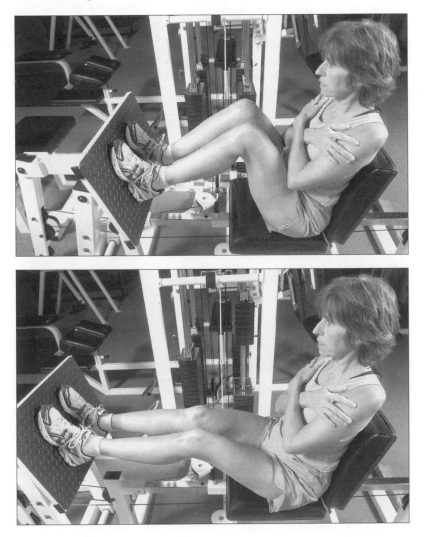

LUNGE

Works the thighs and buttocks

Starting position: Begin with your feet a little wider than shoulder-width apart. Make sure you have adequate open space in front of you.

Front Lunge Movement: Step forward with your right leg (about two to three normal step lengths). Slowly drop your left knee toward the floor (stop at about one to two inches above the floor) as you bend your right knee. Your right knee should be directly over your right foot so that your upper and lower leg are at a 90-degree angle. If your knee extends past your foot, you have not stepped out far enough and should adjust accordingly on the next repetition. Slowly push back up into the starting position. In the beginning, this sequence of movements may seem a bit jerky, but as you build strength and balance, you should be able to do the lunge in one fluid movement. To help maintain your balance, extend your arms out to your sides or use a chair placed against a wall to steady yourself. You can either alternate legs during your set or do all the reps for your right leg and then repeat for your left leg (the latter sequence is a little harder).

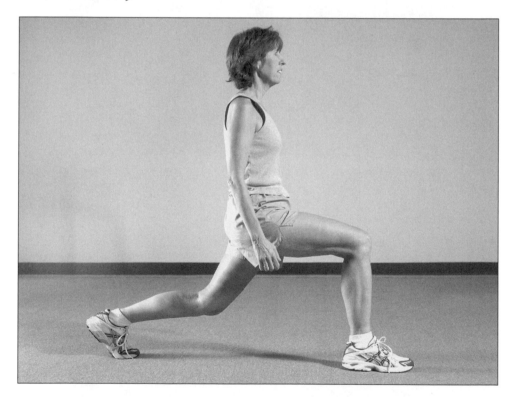

Side Lunge Movement: Rather than stepping forward, step your right leg out to the side and bend your right knee until it is at a 45- to 90-degree angle. Keep your left leg relatively straight and your buttocks stuck out. Be sure to continue facing forward; if you turn and look to your right, you'll just be doing a front lunge. Return to the starting position. Repeat with your left leg.

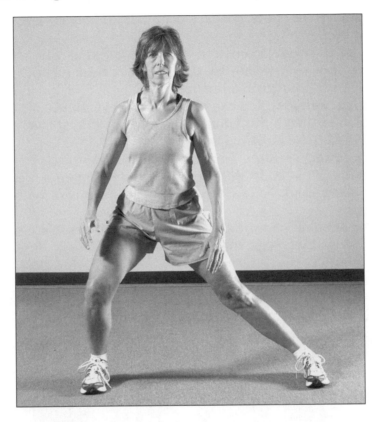

Back Lunge Movement: Rather than stepping forward, step your right leg behind you about two to three step lengths as you bend your left leg to a 45- to 90-degree angle. Keep your back straight throughout the movement. Slowly return to the starting position. Repeat with the left leg. *Note:* This is a very challenging exercise and requires great strength and balance. You should only add it to your program if you have been resistance training for at least three months.

Free-weight version: You can do these same exercises holding a dumbbell in each hand. Since free weights are more challenging for maintaining balance, you should have experience doing these movements and begin with very light weight. A weighted vest is a perfect way to make the front lunge or side lunge more challenging.

Machine version: For the front lunge, a hip flexion and extension machine works similar muscle groups. For the side lunge, a hip abductor machine works similar muscle groups. There is no machine equivalent for the back lunge.

HEEL-TOE RAISE

Works the lower leg

Starting position: Begin with your feet a little wider than shoulder-width apart. You may need to use the back of a chair for balance until you build more strength.

Movement: Slowly raise up onto your toes and then slowly drop your heels. Next, slowly raise your toes as you rock back on your heels and then slowly drop your toes to the floor.

Free-weight version: You can do this same exercise holding a dumbbell in each hand, resting at your sides. A weighted vest is a perfect way to make this exercise more challenging.

Band or tubing version: You can do this same exercise by stepping on the middle of the band with both feet and grasping the ends of the band with each hand. Follow the movement described for the regular heel-toe raise.

Machine version: There is a machine version of this exercise, and you can also do it on a leg press machine (ask your fitness professional for a demonstration).

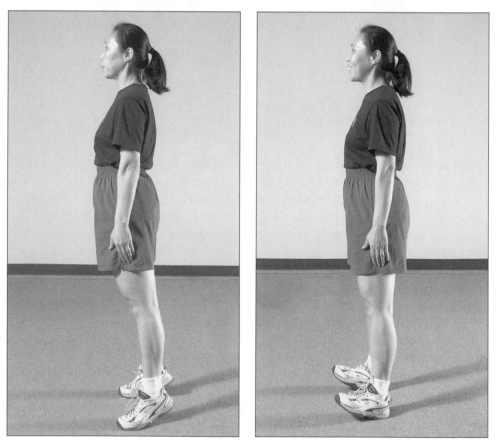

Proper Resistance Exercise Technique

1. Warm up dynamically before resistance exercise (walking, cycling, marching in place) and cool down with stretching.
2. Don't hold your breath!
    ▸ Exhale when you are in the active phase and moving the weight against resistance.
    ▸ Inhale when you are in the recovery phase and moving the weight without resistance.
3. Maintain proper form at all times.
    ▸ Check your form in a mirror.
    ▸ Your set should end if you cannot do any more reps with proper form.
    ▸ You may need to decrease the weight if you cannot maintain form.
4. Move weight or other resistance equipment (band, tubing) slowly for a count of three in each direction.
5. Self-monitor intensity regularly. Adjust the resistance downward if you cannot lift the minimum number of reps or adjust upward if you can lift more than the upper range of reps.
6. Stop exercising if you feel unusual shortness of breath or pain.

Arranging Your Resistance Workout

For any given workout, you can select one or two exercises for each muscle group. Rotate exercises from session to session to provide variety. Do exercises for larger muscle groups first, or those that use many muscles at once, followed by exercises for smaller muscle groups or those that use only one muscle group. A few sample workouts are given in tables 7.1 and 7.2 on page 116. The workouts in table 7.1 include both upper and lower body exercises.

As you progress in your resistance training, or if you have limited time, you may want to do your upper and lower body exercise on separate days (see the sample program in table 7.2). With this type of program, you need to do each workout twice a week, for a total of four workouts per week, to produce optimal benefits. Thus, you may work out for less time per session but more often each week.

Table 7.1   Combined Upper and Lower Body Workouts

Workout A	Workout B
Push-up (regular, bent knee, or wall)	Push-up (regular, bent knee, or wall)
Chest press	Chest fly
One-arm row	Seated row
Upright row	Arm pull-down
Side shoulder raise	Front shoulder raise
Squat or leg press	Chair raise or leg press
Front lunge or hip extension/flexion machine	Side lunge or adductor machine
Step-up	Heel-toe raise

Table 7.2   Separate Upper and Lower Body Workouts

Upper-body workout	Lower-body workout
Push-up	Squat and/or leg press
Chest press	Side lunge or adductor machine
Chest fly	Front lunge or hip extension/flexion machine
One-arm row and/or seated row	Step-up
Arm pull-down and/or side shoulder raise	Heel-toe raise
Single- and/or double-arm biceps curl	
Single-arm triceps extension and/or triceps dip	

Impact Exercise

As noted earlier, impact exercise can be done at home or at a gym, with minimum or more extensive equipment, alone or as a group or sport activity (aerobic dance, volleyball, basketball), indoors or outdoors. In fact, the simplest form of impact exercise, jumping, can be done in a short time period and often without equipment. Chapter 6 includes sample beginning and intermediate jump training programs.

Even though jumping seems rather simple, you can ensure optimum effectiveness and safety by following the tips in the sidebar on page 117. It is easy to slip into poor form when you are tired, so if you find yourself doing this, you may need to lower the intensity of your jumps or stop altogether. Following are examples of proper jump form for a two-foot and one-foot jump.

Proper Jump Technique

▸ Make sure you start with a base of leg strength. If you are a new exerciser, start with three months of resistance exercise before adding jumps.

▸ Always wear stable footwear when jumping (athletic shoes are recommended).

▸ Always jump on a stable, even surface.

▸ If adding jumping to another workout, you may want to do your jumps right after your warm-up when you may be less tired and less prone to accidents. If jumps are added at the end, watch your form and stop if you start to slip out of form!

▸ Land with a slight bend in your knees and your feet flat. *Do not land with your legs completely straight and your knees locked.*

▸ If you feel pain at any point in the jump, including landing, stop. You may need to stop jumping for a week or two (continue to do strengthening exercise if it does not cause pain) and then gradually reintroduce jumping on a limited basis until you can resume your regular routine.

TWO-FOOT JUMP

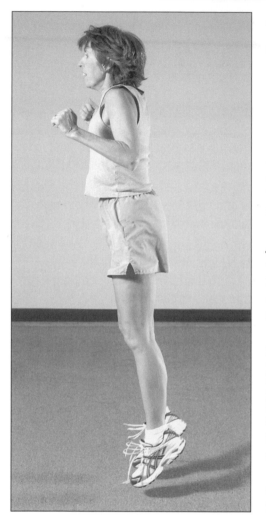

Starting position: Begin with your feet a little wider than shoulder-width apart. Keep your knees slightly bent and your back straight.

Movement: Swing your arms behind you as you bend your knees and then swing your arms forward as you jump into the air (all in one motion). Land straight down in the same place as you lifted off from with both feet flat and a slight bend in your knees.

Line jump (a shortened broad jump): For variation, you can also do these jumps moving forward in a continuous line if you have obstacle-free space. This is fun to do outdoors.

Added height: To increase the intensity of your jump, you could jump onto a bench or step and then jump back off. Some people like to jump forward onto the bench or step and continue in the same direction as they jump off, then turn around for the next jump.

Side jump: You could also jump onto the bench from the side and then jump off to the opposite side, then repeat going the other direction.

Weighted-vest version: To increase the intensity of your jump, you could jump wearing a weighted vest. Remember that you should have built up a base of leg strength before adding a weighted vest to your jumps, and your vest weight for jumps should be about a third to a half of your vest weight for squats or lunges.

ONE-FOOT JUMP

Starting position: Begin with your feet shoulder-width apart and one foot slightly off the floor.

Movement: Bring your arms back a little as you bend your knee slightly, then swing your arms forward (just a little) as you jump into the air, all in one motion. Land with your foot flat and your knee slightly bent.

Side hops: You can start with your right foot up and then push off with your left leg and land on your right foot with your left foot raised. Repeat in the other direction.

Added height: I do not recommend doing one-foot jumps onto and off of a bench or step.

Weighted-vest version: To increase the intensity of your jump, you could jump wearing a weighted vest. Remember that you should have built up a base of leg strength before adding a weighted vest to your jumps, and your vest weight for jumps should be about one-third to half of your vest weight for squats or lunges.

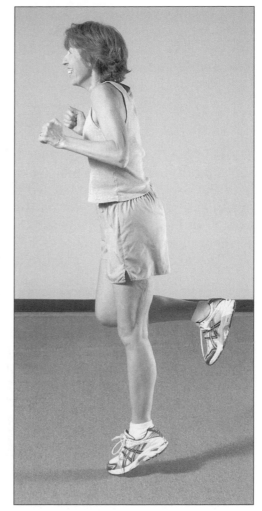

Balance Exercise

Several of the standing versions of the lower body exercises described previously also challenge your balance and thus get two birds with one stone! However, you could add a few specific balance exercises to your program to help improve your balance while standing and walking. Because these exercises are not particularly taxing, you could do them every day.

ONE-LEG STANCE

Starting position: Begin with your feet shoulder-width apart and one foot slightly off the floor. You may feel more secure if you begin by holding onto the back of a straight-backed chair.

Movement: Raise one foot off the floor so that the knee is slightly in front and the foot a few inches off the ground. Hold the position for up to 30 seconds and then switch legs. Repeat up to three to five times on each leg. To make this movement more challenging, close your eyes.

TANDEM (HEEL-TO-TOE) WALK

Starting position: Begin with the heel of your right foot directly in front of your left toes so that your heel and toes are touching. You may feel more secure if you begin by touching a wall.

Movement: Walk forward and bring your left foot directly in front of your right so that the heel of your left foot touches the tip of your right toes. Continue with this heel-to-toe pattern for up to 20 feet. Repeat this walk three to five times.

Stretching Exercises

Stretching, or flexibility exercise, can be done at home or at a gym, with no equipment, indoors or outdoors. Stretching should be a part of every exercise program. To make gains in flexibility, you should do most of your stretching after you exercise, when your muscles are warm and pliable. Each stretch should be held from 10 to 60 seconds and repeated three to five times. To progress your flexibility training, hold a stretch longer or do more repetitions. There are dozens and dozens of stretching exercises, but I describe only a few key exercises here that stretch major muscle groups. If you work a particular muscle group more than others or feel less flexible in a certain area, you may need to add more specific stretches.

Proper Stretching Technique

▸ Go into a stretch relaxed. Don't tense your muscles.

▸ With most stretches, your back should be kept straight. To do this, bend at the hip. *Do not* arch your back and drop your head forward.

▸ Most stretches are done "statically," meaning you do not bounce or jerk during the stretch, but hold it for a given duration. If a stretch is done in motion, the movement should be slow and gradual, not "ballistic."

▸ In seated stretches, do not lock your knees when your legs are extended. Keep your knees slightly bent.

▸ You should "feel" the stretch but not pain. If you feel *any* pain, back off slightly until it subsides. If you can't do a stretch without pain, don't do it.

▸ If you have osteoporosis, do not hyperextend your spine (lie on your belly and raise your chest far off the floor).

STANDING THIGH STRETCH

Starting position: Stand with your feet shoulder-width apart. You may feel more comfortable with your nonexercising hand holding a wall or the back of a straight-backed chair.

Movement: Bend your left leg back at the knee and grasp your left ankle. Keep your left leg parallel to your standing (right) leg and your knees close together. You may need to push your knee back slightly to feel the stretch. You should feel the stretch along the front of your thigh. Repeat with the right leg.

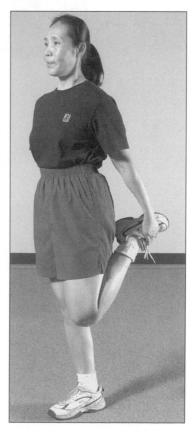

SEATED HAMSTRING STRETCH

Note: **This is similar to the sit-and-reach test.**

Starting position: Sit near the edge of a stable, straight-backed chair with your right leg extended out in front (slightly bent at the knee) and your right foot flexed back. Your left knee should be bent with your left foot flat on the floor, aligned directly under your knee.

Movement: Bending at the waist, slowly extend your arms forward, parallel to your outstretched leg, and toward your right foot. Move forward until you feel a stretch along the back of your right leg and hold. Repeat with the left leg.

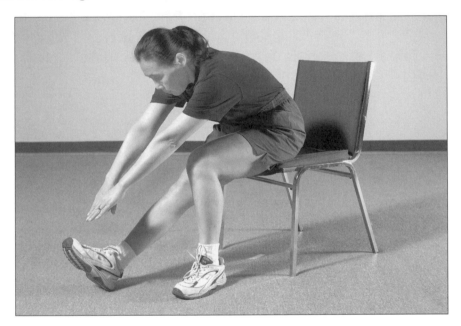

STANDING CALF STRETCH

Starting position: Stand facing a wall with your feet shoulder-width apart. Step your left foot forward, just in front of the wall, with the knee slightly bent. Step your right foot back and drop your heel to the floor. Place your forearms flat against the wall with your palms on the wall.

Movement: Lean forward toward the wall, keeping both feet flat on the floor. You should feel the stretch along your right calf. If you do not feel the stretch, lean in farther toward the wall and try to bend your right knee a little more. You could also step your right leg back a few inches and lean in again. Repeat with the other leg.

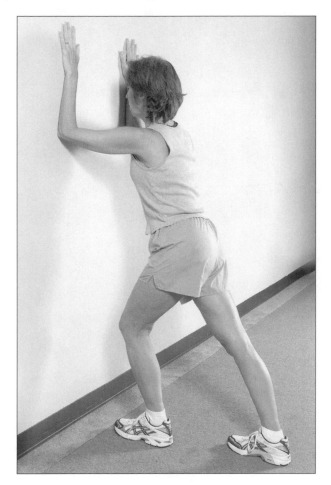

DOORWAY CHEST STRETCH

Starting position: Standing in the middle of a doorway, raise your arms, keeping them bent at the elbow, and rest your lower arm and hands flat against each side of the door.

Movement: Slowly lean forward with your chest, keeping your feet flat on the floor. You should feel the stretch along your chest and the front of your shoulders.

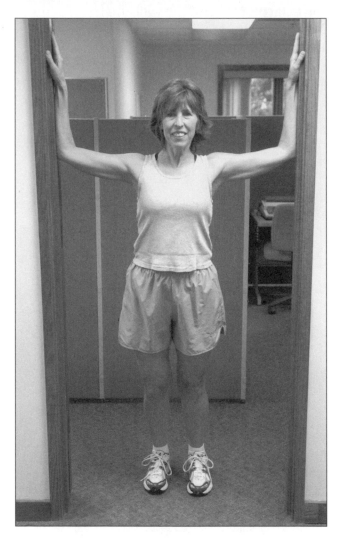

SHOULDER STRETCH

Starting position: Stand or sit with your right arm wrapped across your chest and hold it against your chest with your left hand.

    Movement: With your left hand, gently press your right arm closer to and slightly across your chest to feel a stretch along your right shoulder. Repeat with the other arm.

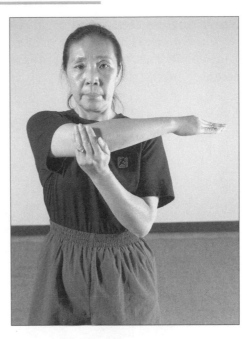

TRICEPS STRETCH

Starting position: Stand or sit and raise your right arm over your head, then bend at the elbow so that your hand is touching the back of your shoulders (your elbow should be pointed straight in the air).

    Movement: Gently push your elbow down with your left hand until you feel a stretch along the back of your upper arm. Repeat on the other side.

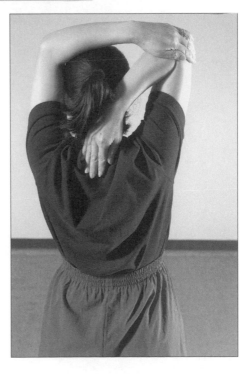

NECK STRETCH

Starting position: Stand or sit with your shoulders relaxed.

    Movement: Gently drop your right ear toward your right shoulder so that you feel a stretch along the left side of your neck. Repeat to the other side.

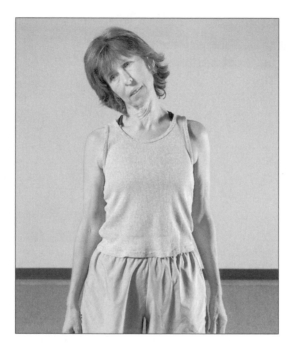

Summary

Any exercise program must address important elements of the plan that will ensure you are doing exercises properly for your safety and for optimal benefit. Exercise can be done in many settings, and each has its advantages and disadvantages. Consider these when planning where to exercise, but remain flexible and seek alternative options if your current setting is not working for you. Equipment is essential for any exercise program; costs can range from minimal to extensive, and this may determine what type of exercise you do and where you do it. Proper equipment can also help promote safety, so try not to neglect this important area. Proper form is the hallmark of safety and effectiveness for any type of exercise, so be sure you know what proper form is and avoid losing form when you become tired. You may want to seek help from an exercise professional to learn proper form initially, although you need not do so to begin an exercise program.

ACTION PLAN:
BENEFITING FROM PROPER TECHNIQUE

- ☐ Determine where you will exercise and what type of equipment you will need.
- ☐ Review the selected exercises for each type of activity: aerobic, resistance, impact, balance, and flexibility.
- ☐ Choose exercises that will best meet your goals and, using the information in chapter 6, design a four-week program.
- ☐ Keep in mind the tips and techniques for safe and effective exercise outlined in this chapter.

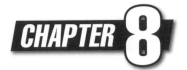
MAKING WISE NUTRITIONAL CHOICES

The quality of your diet can influence the health of your bones. Most of us know that taking in enough calcium is an important factor in bone health. Fewer of us know that other nutrients have the potential to influence the strength of our skeleton. In this chapter, I discuss the important nutrients that can help or harm your bones and make recommendations for how to improve your diet to optimize your bone health. I also discuss the role of nutritional supplements in achieving your health goals.

As explained in chapter 1, calcium is a critical nutrient for bone health and for many other important bodily functions such as nerve transmission, blood clotting, chemical signaling, and muscle contraction. The body ardently defends its blood levels of calcium, which are challenged each day by usual losses through skin shedding, nail loss, sweat, and bladder or bowel elimination. If the body does not replace its daily losses through diet, it keeps blood levels steady by taking calcium from the bones. In addition to dietary deficiency of calcium, some dietary habits cause greater than usual calcium losses from the body (increased urinary excretion). Additionally, getting the calcium from nutrients into the bloodstream may be problematic (impaired absorption). Increases in calcium loss or decreases in calcium absorption can cause the skeleton to forfeit some of its stores to keep blood levels normal. Many other dietary substances help keep bones healthy and blood calcium normal (U.S. Department of Health and Human Services 2004).

The well-known cliché "everything in moderation" applies to the dietary recommendations aimed at boosting your bone health. Research has shown that too little or too much of several nutrients may be bad for your bones and may increase the fracture risk. As with other dietary recommendations, a healthy, well-balanced diet should provide the necessary building blocks for healthy bones. Even with the best efforts, however, our diets may fall short of meeting recommended levels. In this case, dietary supplements may help you get the necessary amounts of important nutrients. Be aware, however, that supplements should only be used to help you *meet* recommended dietary levels. An increasingly popular trend is to "megadose" on vitamins based on the notion that "if some is good, more is better." With respect to nutrients, this adage is not necessarily true and in several cases can actually be harmful. Extremely high amounts of some nutrients can have adverse health effects, often quite serious. Dietary supplements are not medicine and should be used wisely and only when necessary.

A Bone-Healthy Diet

In a recent conversation about nutritional supplements, a colleague asked, "Well, how do I know if I need to supplement my diet?" I told her she had asked a very smart question, and we discussed some options. Obviously, you could consult with a registered dietician, who is a licensed professional trained to evaluate your diet and help you develop and adopt sound nutritional habits. Although ideal, this means of evaluating and revising your diet could be cost-prohibitive. Registered dieticians are the only nutrition professionals that have a college degree, have specialized training, and have passed a national board exam to ensure their credibility. If you cannot afford to consult with a registered dietician, there are simpler ways to evaluate your diet.

The simplest way to tell if you are getting enough or too much of certain nutrients is to keep a log of everything you eat and drink for a few days. You need to be as honest and accurate as possible, keeping track of both what and how much you eat and drink. To tell how much of a particular nutrient you consume on an average day, you have to find the nutrient values for each food and add them up for the day. If you keep a diet record for more than one day, you have to calculate the average nutrient levels per day. Obviously, determining nutrient values for mixed foods such as casseroles and sweets can be difficult. Nutrient values can be found in many nutrition books and now commonly on the Internet. There are even free programs on the Internet that will calculate the nutrient composition of your diet if you enter the amount and types of food or drink you've consumed. Tables 8.2 through 8.6 list the nutrient values for some common foods that are high in bone-related nutrients, but be aware that this is only a small selection of foods. Comparing your diet to these lists, however, could reflect whether you are consuming foods known to be rich in nutrients. A diet log will only give you a general estimate of your nutrient intake, but taking even a general look at what you are eating can give you some idea about the quality of your diet.

Vitamins and Minerals

Vitamins and minerals are substances the body needs for normal growth, repair, and function. The body must acquire most of these nutrients from the diet. Although many vitamins and minerals play a role in bone health, I've focused on the few that research suggests are the most important and those that are often too low or too high in the typical Western diet.

Calcium

Nearly everyone knows that calcium is important for strong bones. We learned this when we were kids, and we have been reminded again in recent years by dozens of billboards and magazine ads of celebrities with milk moustaches urging us to drink milk. Calcium is the most essential building block for your bones. It combines with other minerals to form the hard crystals that give bone its strength. When our supply of dietary calcium is insufficient, some of these crystals dissolve and give their calcium back to the bloodstream. Because our bodies cannot make calcium, it *must* come from our diets. Research has shown that people in countries that have greater milk consumption have fewer fractures and those in countries that don't consume much milk or dairy products tend to have more fractures. So how much calcium must we take in to keep our bones strong?

Determining the Proper Amount of Calcium

Extensive research has been done to help determine the optimal calcium intake for keeping our bones healthy. Humans are pretty poor calcium absorbers, so we have to ingest a lot of calcium just to offset the small bodily calcium loss each day. As we get older, our ability to absorb calcium tends to get worse, so our dietary calcium requirement increases. To prevent bone loss, recommended dietary intakes of calcium for adult women aged 19 to 50 years is 1,000 milligrams per day. This increases slightly to 1,200 milligrams per day for men and women over 50 (Institute of Medicine Food and Nutrition Board 1997). These recommended intakes are equivalent to the calcium ingested from three to four cups of milk or two to three cups of yogurt per day.

The abundant research on dietary calcium and bone health suggests that the optimal time for calcium to improve bone growth is during the growing years. If you have daughters or granddaughters of this age, it is vital that they get as much calcium in their diet as possible because it can make for significantly improved bone health when they are adults. For adults, the role of dietary calcium is preventing bone loss. Studies show that calcium intakes at or above recommended levels don't necessarily *increase* bone density but are important in preventing bone loss over time. This is especially true for people who habitually consume less than half the recommended level of calcium. Unfortunately, many American women fall into this category (Fleming and Heimbach 1994). You would be wise to assess the amount of calcium in your diet.

Some people, particularly those with low bone density or a family history of osteoporosis, are very determined to get enough calcium in their diet. Many of them, however, are frustrated to learn that their diligent attention to increasing the calcium in their diet does not increase their bone density. Calcium is not a magic pill, but it is an important mineral for bone health that must be adequate in the diet or bone loss will worsen. Adequate calcium intake is *one* important part of a comprehensive strategy to keep your bones healthy. The next section includes suggestions on how to improve the calcium content of your diet naturally through foods or, if needed, through supplements. *Note:* Excessive calcium intakes can contribute to kidney stone formation in certain individuals. Intakes above 2,500 milligrams per day should be avoided.

Improving the Calcium in Your Diet

As with all nutrients, calcium is most usable by the body when ingested in the form of food. We know that dairy products such as milk, yogurt, and cheese are high in calcium. Foods such as nuts, fish, beans, and some vegetables contain less calcium but can help round out your intake of dairy products to achieve your calcium requirement. Because calcium is such an important nutrient in our diet, many nondairy foods, such as orange juice, bread, cereals, and even margarine, are fortified with calcium. Be sure to read how much extra calcium per serving these fortified foods contain, because some (calcium-fortified margarine, for example) contain rather paltry amounts. See table 8.1 for the calcium content of selected foods.

People often find it difficult to consume their daily requirement of calcium in the form of food. Some have trouble digesting lactose (lactose maldigestion or lactose intolerance), the sugar in milk, and find that dairy-based foods upset their stomach. Others find it difficult to eat enough calcium-rich foods. For those with lactose maldigestion or lactose intolerance, some dairy-based foods such as yogurt cause less discomfort. Lactose pills taken before consumption of dairy-based foods or added to foods can curtail gastrointestinal symptoms. If you have lactose intolerance or do not otherwise consume enough dairy products, calcium supplements may help you achieve your daily requirement.

Calcium Supplements

Calcium supplements come in many forms and are a good way to take in extra calcium. Calcium supplements can be in the form of calcium phosphate, calcium carbonate, and calcium citrate, which are all fine sources. They may be taken in pill, chewable, or liquid form. Personally, I like the chewable and liquid forms because I find the large calcium pills hard to swallow. Not all of the calcium in a supplement is available to the body, so

Table 8.1 Calcium Content of Selected Foods

Food	Amount	Calcium (mg)
Milk (reduced fat 2%)	1 cup	270
Yogurt (nonfat, plain)	1 cup	450
Hard cheese (cheddar)	1 oz	200
Cottage cheese (lowfat)	1 cup	150
Ice cream (vanilla)	1 cup	84
Tofu (soybean curd; firm)	¼ block	130
Nuts (almonds)	1 oz (24 nuts)	70
Beans (navy)	1 cup cooked	130
Sardines with bones	3 oz canned	325
Molasses, blackstrap	1 tbsp.	175
Spinach	1 cup raw	30
Broccoli	1/2 cup cooked	30
Orange	1 medium, raw	50

be sure to base your dosage on the *elemental* amount of calcium in each pill. If the elemental calcium is not listed on the label, you must assume that the calcium is in the elemental form. Calcium supplements are often packaged with other vitamins and minerals (e.g., vitamin D, magnesium, and zinc) and sold as "bone-wise" combinations or similar packages. Unless you know you are deficient in these other nutrients, you don't need to take these combination supplements.

The stomach can only absorb about 500 milligrams of calcium at a time. Any more than that gets excreted, so it is best to spread your supplement ingestion throughout the day. For example, if you take 1,000 milligrams per day, you should take 500 milligrams in the morning and 500 milligrams in the evening. Some people may experience gastrointestinal distress (cramping, diarrhea, discomfort) from supplements. If you experience these symptoms, you should try a different form or type of supplement because they may cause fewer symptoms. If you've never taken supplements, begin by taking small amounts and increase your intake gradually.

A wide variety of supplement brands are available, and you want to be sure you are taking one that is safe and effective. Supplements made from bone meal, dolomite, or unrefined oyster shells should be avoided because they may contain substances such as lead or other toxic metals that come out in the process of extracting calcium. To help ensure that the supplement you are taking is safe and effective, look for products that have AUSP@ on the label. This label means that the supplement has met voluntary quality standards established by the United States Pharmacopeia (USP) and is less likely to contain harmful contaminants and more likely to disintegrate in the stomach.

Vitamin D

Vitamin D is another important nutrient for bone health because it helps calcium get from the stomach to the bloodstream and then to the bones. Research suggests that low vitamin D levels are related to low bone density and increased risk of fracture (U.S. Department of Health and Human Services 2004). New evidence points to a link between low vitamin D and falls. The recommended daily intake of vitamin D is between 400 and 800 international units (IU). Extra vitamin D is stored in fat tissue and can accumulate if taken in excessive amounts. Intakes in excess of 800 IU per day are unnecessary unless prescribed by your doctor, and massive doses of vitamin D can be harmful.

Vitamin D can be obtained from vitamin D-fortified foods and sunlight. Foods rich in vitamin D include eggs, fatty fish, and cereal and milk fortified with vitamin D (see table 8.2). When UV rays from the sun make contact with the skin, vitamin D is synthesized. Minimal sun exposure (feet, hands, face) of about 15 to 20 minutes per day is usually enough to get most of the needed vitamin D. Sunscreen can reduce vitamin D synthesis by the skin. People may be at risk for vitamin D deficiency if they are housebound, reside in extreme northern latitudes (where seasonally the sun may not be strong enough to synthesize vitamin D), do not consume vitamin D-fortified foods, or have a kidney or liver disorder that interferes with normal vitamin D metabolism.

Vitamin K

Vitamin K is important for normal blood clotting and bone development. Vitamin K deficiency has been linked to lower bone density, but

Table 8.2   *Vitamin D Levels in Selected Foods*

Food	Amount	Vitamin D (IU)
Eggs	1 hard cooked	20
Salmon	3.5 oz cooked	360
Ready-to-eat fortified cereal	3/4-1 cup	40
Milk (nonfat, lowfat, or whole milk)	1 cup	98

incidences of this deficiency are rather uncommon. Recommended levels of vitamin K are 80 micrograms per day for men age 25 and over and 65 micrograms per day for women age 25 and over. Bacteria in our gastrointestinal tract produce about half of the vitamin K we need, and we get the rest from our diet. Table 8.3 is a list of the vitamin K levels for several foods rich in vitamin K. Vitamin K supplementation is generally unnecessary for most people and could be harmful for those on blood-thinning medications.

Table 8.3   Vitamin K Levels in Selected Foods

Food	Serving size	Vitamin K (μg)
Spinach	1 cup raw	120
Kale	1 cup raw	547
Swiss chard	1 cup raw	299
Green leaf lettuce	1 cup raw	97
Blackberries	1 cup	29

Vitamin A

Vitamin A is important for healthy vision, healthy skin, reproduction, and growth. Vitamin A comes in two forms: retinol and beta-carotene. Retinol is the form that has biologic activity, and beta-carotene is the form that can later be made into retinol. High levels of vitamin A in the form of retinol have been linked to an *increased* risk of fractures (Michaelsson et al. 2003). Precisely how high vitamin A may cause more fractures is unclear, but it is probably prudent to avoid taking vitamin A supplements if you have marginal to poor bone health. Most individuals will get the proper amount of vitamin A through a normal, balanced diet. Recommended dietary levels of vitamin A are 2,300 IU for women and 3,000 IU for men, also expressed in retinol equivalents (RE) of 800 μgRE and 1,000 μgRE for women and men, respectively. The Institute of Medicine warns against consuming more than 10,000 IU of vitamin A daily. Most cases of excessive vitamin A intake occur in older adults who use vitamin supplements. A well-balanced diet is unlikely to lead to excessively high levels of vitamin A. Foods rich in vitamin A include dark, leafy green vegetables, rich yellow or deep-orange vegetables and fruits (e.g., winter squash, carrots, yellow peppers, cantaloupe), milk, cheese, butter, and eggs. The vitamin A content of these foods is listed in table 8.4.

Table 8.4   Vitamin A Levels in Selected Foods

Food	Amount	Vitamin A (µgRE)
Spinach	1 cup raw	375
Carrot	1/2 cup shredded raw	1,100
Mango	1	800
Milk (nonfat, lowfat, whole)	1 cup	130
Eggs	1 hard cooked	80
Cheddar cheese	1.5 oz	130

Sodium

Sodium is important for normal water balance, acid-base balance, nerve transmission, and muscle contraction. As most of us know, excess sodium has been linked to high blood pressure. Recently, excess sodium has also been linked to increased calcium loss from the body (through urinary losses), but the overall research on this topic is inconclusive. Since nearly all processed foods and many whole foods contain sodium, we are usually concerned with limiting our sodium intake rather than increasing it. For overall health, you should try to limit the sodium in your diet to recommended levels. The recommended upper daily intake of sodium is 2,400 milligrams per day. The sodium content of most foods is listed on the nutrition label, so you can easily determine whether you are consuming a food high in sodium. Common high-sodium foods include snack items such as chips and pretzels, condiments, cheese, pickled foods, salty or smoked meats or fish, and canned foods such as soup or cooked vegetables. If your calcium intake is low, you should not exceed recommended levels of sodium intake. Low-sodium alternatives for several high-sodium foods are now available.

Phosphorous

Phosphorous is an important mineral for energy production, cell structure, and bone development. Excess phosphorous has been suspected of reducing calcium absorption, but the scientific evidence for this premise is weak. Recommended intakes of phosphorous are 700 milligrams per day for adults and should not exceed 4,000 milligrams per day. Phosphorous intakes in Western diets have increased over time since phosphorous is abundant in processed foods and cola beverages. If your calcium intake is low, limiting your consumption of high-phosphorous foods may be wise.

Macronutrients

Macronutrients are the large nutrient building blocks of carbohydrate, protein, and fat. These building blocks combine with those from vitamins and minerals to make body cells and maintain function. Of the macronutrients, only protein has been linked to bone health and will be the only one discussed. In line with general dietary recommendations, carbohydrates should make up about 50 to 60 percent of total calorie intake and fats no more than 30 percent.

Both inadequate and excessive protein levels are linked to poor bone health. Protein is an important nutrient for bone because it is the main component of collagen, the substance that gives bone some of its flexibility. It is also the place where the bone mineral embeds itself. Bone cannot be a completely rigid material or it would break from any applied force. Think about what would happen to the frame and chassis of a car if the jolts from every bump and pothole were not lessened somewhat by the shock absorbers. Protein insufficiency, as can occur in older adults who do not consume enough calories, can lessen the shock-absorbing capacity of bone and make it more brittle. Low protein can also reduce the surface area for bone mineral deposits. Both of these factors may underlie observations that people who are protein deficient are more likely to fracture.

Although low protein levels may be harmful to bones, so may high protein levels. Excessive amounts of protein are associated with poor bone health because they can cause more calcium to be excreted from the body by the kidneys. When calcium excretion increases, calcium may be robbed from the bones to offset these losses. The impact of the latest craze of high-protein diets on bone health is yet to be determined, but the implications are not favorable. If you are on a high-protein diet for weight loss, take extra care that you are consuming the daily requirement for calcium and perhaps an additional 100 to 200 milligrams per day.

How much protein is enough and how much is too much? The USDA recommends that average daily protein intake range from 10 percent to 35 percent of total calories consumed (this comes to about 56 grams of protein for an average woman). Most food labels list the percent of calories from protein based on recommendations for a 2000-calorie per day diet. To figure out the percentage of protein in any food, multiply the grams of protein per serving from the food label by 4, divide that by the total number of calories per serving, and multiply the result by 100. Most Americans are believed to exceed the recommended intake for protein in averaged-sized individuals.

All foods are labeled with the protein content per serving, so you can keep a food diary for a day or two and easily determine how much protein you are taking in. For a quick reference, see table 8.5 for the protein content of common foods.

Table 8.5   Protein Content of Selected Foods

Food	Amount	Protein (g)
Meat (steak)	4 oz	50
Fish (broiled salmon)	4 oz	20
Fish (water-packed tuna)	1 cup	40
Chicken (roasted)	1 cup	60
Eggs	1 hard cooked	6
Nuts (almonds)	1 oz (24 nuts)	6
Beans (navy)	1 cup cooked	15
Milk (nonfat, lowfat, whole)	1 cup	8
Yogurt (nonfat, plain)	1 cup	13
Hard cheese	1 oz	7
Cottage cheese (lowfat)	1 cup	31
Fruit (banana)	1 medium	1.5
Vegetables (carrot)	1 cup cooked	1.2

Other Dietary Factors

Other types of foods or compounds in foods may have bone-healthy or bone-harming effects. The research on these other dietary factors is still accumulating, but I've summarized what is generally recommended for bone health. Similar to recommendations for the dietary nutrients listed earlier, moderation is key to minimizing harmful effects. Overindulgence in potentially bone-healthy foods or food compounds should also be avoided until the research is more conclusive.

Phytoestrogens

Phytoestrogens are dietary compounds that have mild estrogenlike activity in the body and have thus been touted as "natural estrogens." The amount of estrogen these foods yield is much less than that produced by the body's organs, such as the ovaries, and less than synthetic forms of estrogen found in hormone replacement preparations or oral contraceptives. The most popular phytoestrogens are probably soybeans and soy-containing products. Soy is from a class of phytoestrogens called isoflavones that are also found in chickpeas and legumes. Because the link between estrogen and bone health is quite strong, phytoestrogens have been explored for their bone-boosting potential, and over-the-counter supplements are also available (most contain ipriflavone). Currently, the evidence for the bone-promoting effects of phytoestrogens is conflicting, so consumption of foods high in phytoestrogens or dietary supplements is not yet recommended for improving bone health. Research is currently being conducted on this topic, however, and more definitive recommendations may be forthcoming. Phytoestrogens have been implicated in reduced or increased risk of other estrogen-related diseases such as heart disease and cancer, but the evidence is still unclear. Moderate intake of foods containing phytoestrogens appears to be safe and may provide some relief from menopausal symptoms.

Caffeine

The link between caffeine and bone health is still unclear. Some studies report greater bone loss in women who consume more than three cups of coffee per day, whereas others find no relationship between coffee and bone health. Interestingly, one study reported that adding a tablespoon or two of milk to coffee offset any bone loss related to caffeine. Although coffee may have no direct effect on bone health, it may have an indirect effect because women who drink coffee may be substituting it for milk or milk-based beverages. If you are a coffee consumer, you should take a careful look at your calcium intake. If you find that your consumption of calcium-rich foods is low, you should consider improving your diet or taking a supplement. You may want to add some milk to your coffee too!

Alcohol

The link between alcohol and bone health is also unresolved. Excessive intakes of alcohol may increase the risk of fracture due to low bone density and increased falls. Consumption of large quantities of alcohol is often linked to poor nutrition and low body weight, both risk factors for poor bone health. Excess alcohol consumption can impair stability and vision, increasing the risk of falls. Moderate intakes of alcohol have been linked to higher bone density compared to those who take in large amounts or no alcohol, but the mechanism is unclear. Again, moderation is the key.

Soft Drinks

Another presumed dietary link to low bone density is soft drink consumption, particularly cola-type beverages. People who drink a lot of soft drinks may be less likely to consume adequate amounts of milk-based beverages and thus more likely to be calcium-deficient. Teenage girls are particularly likely to follow such a trend. Since the phosphorous content of cola beverages is high, people who consume these drinks may be more vulnerable to calcium deficiency, particularly if their diet is low in calcium.

Compiling a Healthy Eating Plan

Now that we've covered the nutrients and foods that affect your bone health, how can you pull all this together to meet your bone health goals? Table 8.6 summarizes the important nutrients for bone health and the recommended intakes for each. Remember that following the USDA Food Guide Pyramid (see figure 8.1) is a great way to guide your food choices. A sensible diet that includes a variety of foods, particularly fresh fruits

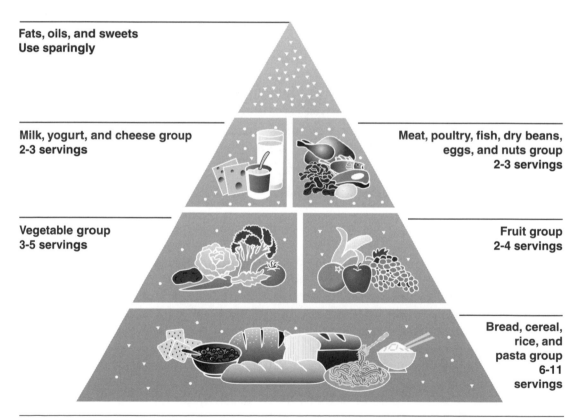

Figure 8.1 USDA Food Guide Pyramid.
Source: U.S. Department of Agriculture/U.S. Department of Health and Human Services.

Table 8.6 Recommended Nutrient and Food Intakes for Bone-Healthy Eating in Adults

Nutrient/food	Recommended daily intake
Calcium	19-50 years: 1,000 51+ years: 1,200
Vitamin D	400-800 international units (IU)
Vitamin K	80 µg/day for men 25 and over and 65 µg/day for women 25 and over
Vitamin A	2,300 IU for women and 3,000 IU for men, or 800 µgRE for women and 1,000 µgRE for men No more than 10,000 IU of vitamin A daily
Sodium	No more than 2,300 mg per day
Phosphorous	700 mg per day for adults, not to exceed 4,000 mg per day
Protein	10-35% of total calories
Carbohydrates and fat	45-65% of total calories from carbohydrates and no more than 20-35% of total calories from fat
Phytoestrogens, caffeine, alcohol, and soft drinks	No recommended amount to aim for or to avoid; moderate intake of these factors is wise

and vegetables, can help ensure adequate vitamin and mineral intake. The proper amounts of calcium may be more difficult to get from produce, so be sure to consume enough dairy products to achieve your recommended intake or consider taking a supplement. Avoiding high amounts of saturated fats, salts, and sugar can ensure that you are not replacing nutrient-dense foods with ones that may be highly processed and low in important nutrients.

Table 8.7 shows an example of modifying an eating plan so that it is more healthful. The first sample menu is a typical day of eating for a 58-year old woman who is 5 feet, 4 inches tall and weighs about 120 pounds. She has borderline osteoporosis at the spine. Her diet is based on convenience foods that are often high in fat and not nutrient dense. By making some healthful modifications to her diet, including adding nonfat dairy products and including more fruits, vegetables, and whole foods, she has reduced her caloric intake and her fat intake and has increased her calcium intake significantly. These simple modifications can help boost the nutritional power of your diet and still keep you satisfied.

Table 8.7 Modifying an Eating Plan for Better Health

For a 58-year-old postmenopausal woman with borderline osteoporosis at the spine; she is 5 feet, 4 inches tall and 120 pounds.

Meal	Original menu	Revised menu
Breakfast	2 cups coffee w/ 2 tsp. sugar 1 large blueberry muffin	1 cup fortified cereal (e.g., Total or Wheaties) 1/2 small banana, sliced 1 cup nonfat milk 1 cup noncaffeinated tea
Midmorning snack	1 powdered doughnut	1 8 oz. carton nonfat flavored yogurt 1 small bagel
Lunch	Caesar salad with grilled chicken and 3 tbsp. dressing 1 slice garlic bread 1 diet cola 1 chocolate chip cookie	2 cups raw spinach salad with 1 hard-boiled egg 1 tbsp. low-fat vinaigrette 1 cup bean soup 3 gingersnap cookies
Afternoon snack	Small bag of potato chips	Small handful (~24) dry-roasted almonds 1 cup carrot and celery sticks 1 tbsp. nonfat ranch dressing
Dinner	Spaghetti with meatballs (1 cup pasta and 3/4 cup marinara sauce with 3 small meatballs) Small dinner salad with 1 tbsp. ranch dressing 1 dinner roll with 2 tsp. butter 1 glass red wine	4 oz. baked or broiled salmon, tuna, or other fatty fish 1 tbsp. nonfat tartar sauce 1 cup steamed broccoli 1/2 cup long-grain rice 1 whole-wheat dinner roll with 1 tsp. butter
Dessert	2 cups microwave popcorn with butter	1 cup nonfat chocolate-flavored instant pudding
Nutritional analysis of sample menu (estimated values)		
	Total calories: 2,304 (recommended is 1,900 per day) Calories from protein: ~10% Calories from fat: ~50% Calories from carbohydrate: ~40% Calcium intake: 235 mg	Total calories: 1,877 Calories from protein: 19% Calories from fat: 27% Calories from carbohydrate: 54% Calcium intake: 1,800 mg

Summary

Proper nutrition is a key component of any program aimed at promoting better bone health. Although calcium and vitamin D are well-recognized as important for bone health, other factors may have additional bone-promoting effects and some may have bone-harming effects. Consuming a well-balanced diet that meets the dietary recommendations is an ideal way to help optimize your bone health. If you suspect you are deficient in a nutrient, over-the-counter supplements may be necessary. Select supplements that are tested for their safety and effectiveness. Moderating your intake of nutrients or compounds that do not help bone can minimize or avoid their adverse effects. You may wish to track what you eat and drink over a few days to get an idea of whether you are consuming the right nutrients in the recommended amounts. Modifying your diet accordingly can help you achieve your plan for good bone health.

ACTION PLAN:

MAKING WISE NUTRITIONAL CHOICES

- ☐ Evaluate your diet by keeping a diet record for a few days.
- ☐ Know how much calcium you should ingest per day.
- ☐ Be aware of other nutrients that play a role in bone health—both those that help and those that harm bone.
- ☐ Eat a well-balanced diet to achieve recommended dietary levels of nutrients important for bone health.
- ☐ Consider supplementation to achieve recommended dietary levels.
- ☐ Reduce consumption of or avoid foods that may increase calcium loss or impair calcium absorption, particularly if your diet is low in calcium.
- ☐ Remember that nutrients are not medicine and should be considered only part of an overall strategy for optimal health.

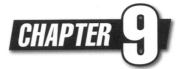

CHAPTER 9

CONSIDERING THE PROS AND CONS OF MEDICATION

For most of you who are diagnosed with osteoporosis, pharmaceutical intervention will be recommended by your physician to reduce your risk of fracture. For some of you with osteopenia, pharmaceutical intervention will be recommended to reduce your risk of developing osteoporosis. If you have osteopenia, the decision on whether to initiate drug intervention may depend on your age and current bone density, how your bone density has changed over time (if the information is available), and your risk factor profile. If these three elements indicate that your risk of developing osteoporosis is substantial and impending, drug and lifestyle intervention may be a wise option. If they indicate that your risk is modest, lifestyle management may be a suitable option for the time being.

Over the past decade, notable advancements have been made in drugs targeted at increasing bone density and reducing fractures. New drugs continue to be developed, and current drugs are being reformulated to improve effectiveness, reduce dosage, and mitigate side effects. Some drugs are more effective than others, and some have more side effects. Your physician is best suited to determine which drug is most appropriate for treating your particular condition and disease stage or threat. However, by informing yourself about the various treatment options, you can work with your physician to find the treatment or prevention program most appropriate for you.

In this chapter, we'll discuss the drugs that are currently approved by the Federal Drug Administration (FDA) for the prevention or treatment of osteoporosis, for whom and for what conditions they are approved, how well they work, and their side effects. You should be aware, however, that although many of these drugs can effectively reduce fracture rates by up to 50 percent, none are 100 percent effective. Thus, you need to consider all of the factors that contribute to fracture risk (i.e., exercise, nutrition, fall risk) to ensure that you follow a comprehensive program that may include drug management. The information contained in this chapter and throughout the text can help you create such a program.

Approved Treatments for Osteoporosis

All of the currently approved drugs reduce fracture rates by increasing bone density and reducing rates of bone turnover. As discussed in chapter 1, bone loss results from either increased bone loss or decreased bone formation. All but one of the currently approved drugs work by reducing the amount of bone lost such that a net gain in bone density occurs over time. The drugs that reduce bone loss render ineffective the bone cells that break down bone. The one drug that forms new bone is thought to stimulate bone-forming cells, but the precise action of this drug is still unknown. The currently approved classes of drugs are categorized as bisphosphonates, estrogen replacement or hormone replacement therapies, selective estrogen receptor modulators (SERMs), and synthetic calcium-regulating hormones (see table 9.1 on page 151). We'll discuss each class of drugs in the following sections.

Bisphosphonates

The class of drugs called bisphosphonates is currently the most effective at reducing osteoporotic fractures. Two forms of bisphosphonates are currently available: alendronate (brand name Fosamax) and risedronate (brand name Actonel). Both drugs reduce fractures by increasing bone density and reducing bone turnover. They do this by rendering the cells that break down bone inactive while leaving the cells that form bone alone. On average, these drugs cause bone density to increase by approximately 4 to 8 percent at the spine and 1 to 3 percent at the hip over the first three to four years of treatment (Black et al. 1996; Cummings et al. 1998; Heaney et al. 2002). Increases in bone density generally plateau at around the fourth year of use, so that continued use of the drug then maintains a higher level of bone density. Both of these drugs have been shown to reduce spine fractures by as much as 40 to 50 percent and hip fractures by as much as 30 to 50 percent (Black et al. 1996, Cummings et al. 1998, Heaney et al. 2002). Currently, because of their potent fracture-reducing ability, bisphosphonates are the most widely prescribed drugs for treating osteoporosis.

Patients taking bisphosphonates often tell me that they expect to be taking the drug indefinitely. I usually tell them that much is still unknown about the long-term use and effectiveness of bisphosphonate therapy, so this should be an ongoing discussion with their physician as long as they take the drug. The longest-running study on alendronate is seven years and shows that the antifracture effects of the drug persist over this time span (Tonino et al. 2000). No study has determined how well alendronate works and whether any side effects occur after more than seven years of treatment. A few studies on women who stopped using bisphosphonates show that bone density remains elevated for the first year after discontinuing the drug. Some very small bone loss may begin thereafter, but not enough to increase fracture risk (Greenspan et al. 2002, Tonino et al. 2000). Thus, the length of time someone must remain on this drug is still uncertain.

Both bisphosphonate drugs are currently approved by the FDA for the treatment of postmenopausal osteoporosis and bone loss in women, bone loss in men, and the treatment of osteoporosis caused by long-term glucocorticoid (i.e., cortisone, prednisone) use. More recently, both drugs were also approved for the prevention of osteoporosis in postmenopausal women at significant risk for developing the disease. Reported side effects of both drugs are few, but include an increased incidence of upper gastro-intestinal distress, heartburn, indigestion, chest discomfort, and pain with swallowing, although risedronate may have a lower rate of these problems (Adachi et al. 2001). Individuals must remain upright for 30 minutes after taking bisphosphonates, and many find this to be inconvenient and bothersome; however, recent reformulations of each drug into once-weekly tablets greatly reduce this problem.

Estrogen Replacement or Hormone Replacement Therapies

Most women are aware that hormone replacement therapies reduce menopausal symptoms (e.g., hot flashes, dry skin) and are beneficial for bone. For many women, hormone replacement therapies have been prescribed specifically to reduce menopause-related bone loss. They offset the estrogen-related bone loss associated with menopause and even cause a slight increase in hip and spine bone density that plateaus after three years of use (Greendale et al. 2002). Studies show that hormone replacement therapies reduce the incidence of fractures of the hip and spine by 30 to 50 percent (Cauley et al. 2003). When they are discontinued, however, bone density is lost, in a manner similar to what occurs in menopause (Greenspan et al. 2002).

Hormone replacement therapies are currently approved for reducing postmenopausal bone loss as a means of preventing osteoporosis but are ineffective at preventing bone loss in men. For bone loss prevention to be most effective, women should begin therapy close to, if not a few years before, the menopausal transition (Bjarnason et al. 2002). Although HRT and ERT are still effective at reducing bone loss if begun several years after menopause, beginning therapy closer to menopause reduces the absolute loss of bone. Estrogen replacement therapy, consisting only of estrogen, is recommended for women who have undergone a hysterectomy and are thus considered postmenopausal. Hormone replacement therapy, consisting of both estrogen and progesterone, is recommended for women who have not had a hysterectomy but have gone through a natural menopause. Women who might become pregnant, have breast cancer or other estrogen-dependent cancer, or have a risk of thromboembolic disease (blood clots in the legs) should not take hormone replacement therapies. Side effects of hormone replacement therapies may include irregular vaginal bleeding (in women who haven't undergone a hysterectomy), fluid retention, headaches, and small but increased risks of abnormal blood clots and breast cancer.

HRT has been touted to have additional health benefits that may protect against heart disease. Higher levels of good cholesterol and lower levels

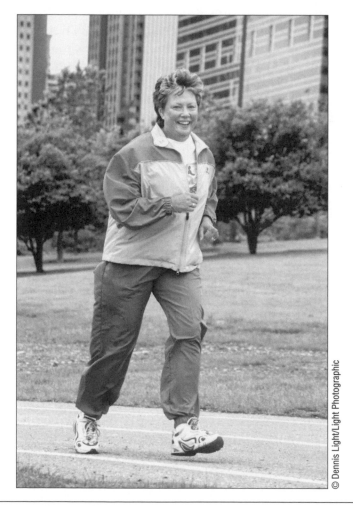

© Dennis Light/Light Photographic

When starting a new medication, check with your doctor about possible reactions of the medication to exercise.

of bad cholesterol were reported in women taking hormone replacement therapies compared to women who did not. Similar studies also reported fewer cardiovascular incidents in women taking hormone replacement therapies compared to those who did not (Knopp et al. 1994). Recently, however, these findings have come under scrutiny. The Women's Health Initiative (WHI), a large clinical research study, was in part designed to specifically examine the health benefits of hormone replacement therapies in women. The study confirmed that these therapies increased bone density in postmenopausal women and effectively lowered the incidence of fractures. However, the study also reported an increase in the number of adverse cardiovascular events (i.e., stroke, heart attack) in women taking hormone replacement therapy compared to those who were not (Cauley et al. 2003, Wassertheil-Smoller et al. 2003). The sponsor of the WHI study, the National Institutes of Health (NIH), was concerned enough by the information that they stopped the trial and released the study findings to the public. The NIH currently sponsors a Web site that addresses questions and concerns about the use of ERT or HRT based on the latest research findings (www.nhlbi.nih.gov/health/women/pht_facts.htm). Recent studies are investigating the use of very low dose estrogen to preserve bone yet minimize the risk of stroke and breast cancer. Topically applied hormone preparations such as progesterone creams have not been shown to have favorable effects on bone but may help alleviate menopausal symptoms (Leonetti et al. 1999).

Selective Estrogen Receptor Modulators

Selective estrogen receptor modulators, or SERMs, are a class of drugs that act in a manner that is either similar to or opposite to estrogen, depending on the body organ the drug is acting on. For example, the cancer drug tamoxifen is used in breast cancer treatment because it acts against estrogen in breast tissue, thereby helping to reduce tumor growth, but tamoxifen acts like estrogen on bone, thereby slowing bone loss. Raloxifene (brand name Evista), a drug similar to tamoxifen, has been approved for reducing bone loss in postmenopausal women because it, too, acts like estrogen on bone.

Recent studies have shown that raloxifene modestly increases spine and hip bone density and reduces bone turnover in postmenopausal women. It reduces spine fractures by up to 50 percent but appears to be less effective at preventing bone loss at the hip and has thus far shown no ability to reduce hip or other nonspine fractures (Ettinger et al. 1999). Raloxifene does not have the same alleviating effect on menopausal symptoms as HRT or ERT does. In experimental trials, women on raloxifene experienced more hot flashes, vaginal bleeding, leg cramps, and leg swelling and had a greater incidence of venous thromboembolic disease compared to women on placebo. However, raloxifene also reduced the incidence of breast cancer in women at high risk for the disease and reduced levels of harmful cholesterol (Cauley et al. 2001). Raloxifene is currently recommended for treatment of postmenopausal osteoporosis and for preventing bone loss in recently menopausal women. The longest-running study of raloxifene has been slightly more than three years, so its safety and ability to continue to reduce spine fractures after three years of use is uncertain.

Synthetic Calcium-Regulating Hormones

Perhaps one of the longest-standing drugs on the market for bone loss is calcitonin (brand names Miacalcin, Calcimar). Calcitonin is a hormone that causes calcium to be taken up from the blood and deposited in the skeleton. Calcitonin is actually a hormone that the body makes naturally, and its purpose is to prevent excessively high levels of blood calcium. The idea behind using calcitonin as a drug is that if it is given in large amounts with additional dietary calcium, it may cause the extra ingested calcium to go straight to the skeleton. Calcitonin used to be given intravenously but resulted in too many side effects. A nasal spray form was developed and is now the most commonly prescribed form, although users may experience some nasal discomfort.

Calcitonin has been approved for the treatment of postmenopausal osteoporosis. Nasal-spray calcitonin results in slight increases in spine bone density and reduces new spine fractures by about 36 percent (Chesnut et al. 2000). Calcitonin does not appear to increase hip bone density or to reduce hip or other nonspine fractures. The longest-running study of calcitonin has been five years, so its safety and ability to continue to reduce spine fractures after five years of use is uncertain.

The newest drug on the market is a synthetic form of another naturally occurring hormone. Parathyroid hormone (PTH; brand name Forteo) helps defend our bodies against low levels of blood calcium by taking calcium from the bones back into the blood. Interestingly, when synthetic versions of PTH are given at regularly spaced intervals, bone is actually gained! How this happens is a bit puzzling, but studies show that, on average, bone density at the spine can increase up to 10 percent in some people. Unfortunately, PTH is not as effective at building hip bone density and in fact results in no change at all (Hodsman et al. 2003). It has not yet been evaluated for its ability to reduce fractures, but the increases in bone density suggest that it is likely effective at reducing spine fractures. Currently, PTH is approved for the prevention of bone loss in men and women with osteoporosis and high risk of fracture. Side effects of the drug include dizziness and leg cramps. Stay tuned for more on this promising osteoporosis treatment.

As with all types of drug therapy, certain factors should be considered when making the decision to begin, continue, or discontinue treatment. First and foremost, all decisions should be made in consultation with your

Table 9.1 FDA-Approved Treatments for Osteoporosis

Drug class	Approved for	Pros	Cons
Bisphosphonates (*Actonel, Fosamax*)	Postmenopausal osteoporosis; postmenopausal bone loss; male bone loss; glucocorticoid-induced osteoporosis	Large increase in bone density at hip and spine; reduces spine and hip fractures by up to 50%	Small risk of upper GI side effects
ERT/HRT (*Estrace, PremPro*)	Postmenopausal bone loss	Modest increase in bone density; reduces spine and hip fractures by up to 30%	Increased risk of cardiovascular events; slight increase in breast cancer risk
SERMs (*Evista*)	Postmenopausal bone loss	Modest increase in spine bone density, preserves hip bone density; reduces spine fractures by up to 50%; reduction in breast cancer and bad cholesterol	No effect on hip fractures
Synthetic hormone: Calcitonin (*Miacalcin, Calcimar*)	Postmenopausal osteoporosis	Modest increase in spine bone density and reduction in spine fractures by up to 36%	No effect on hip bone density or fractures
Synthetic hormone: Parathyroid hormone (*Forteo*)	Men and women with osteoporosis and high risk of fracture	Potentially large increase in spine bone density (8-10%)	Little to no effect on hip bone density; ability to reduce hip or spine fractures not tested

physician and preferably a specialist in osteoporosis. Considerations to keep in mind include the severity of your disease and disease risk (in the case of osteopenic patients), your age, your current health status, your financial and health coverage situation, your risk of adverse events or of suffering side effects, alternative therapies, and your personal comfort with the recommended regimen. Your bone density should also be monitored regularly before and during drug treatment to ensure that the treatment is having the desired effect.

Combined Effects of Exercise and Drug Therapy on Bone

Since exercise is known to have a positive effect on bone, combining exercise with drug therapy could result in an even greater reduction in fracture risk than just drug therapy alone. Few scientific studies of the combined effects of exercise and drug therapy have been done. Some studies have evaluated the combined effects of ERT or HRT plus exercise as well as alendronate plus exercise on bone health in women. Women who take ERT or HRT and exercise may experience greater gains in bone density than women taking either ERT or HRT or exercising only, suggesting some sort of positive interaction between estrogen and exercise on bone. Only a handful of studies on alendronate plus exercise have been done and suggest little additional benefit of exercise to the potent effect of alendronate; however, the number of trials is too few to reach a solid conclusion.

Although falls are an important risk factor for fractures, to our knowledge, no drug therapy has been shown to independently reduce the risk of falls. Since all wrist fractures, nearly all hip fractures, and about half of all spine fractures are associated with a fall, taking measures to reduce fall risk will decrease your risk of fracture beyond the effects of drug therapy. Furthermore, exercise can affect several aspects of your health in addition to bone and falls, so drug therapy should never be considered a substitute or replacement for exercise; rather, drug and exercise therapy combined should be considered part of a comprehensive program for reducing fracture and chronic disease.

Summary

Several drugs have been developed and approved over the past 15 years for the treatment of osteoporosis and the prevention of bone loss. All of the approved drugs increase spine or hip bone density and all except PTH have been shown to significantly reduce spine and hip fractures. The appropriate drug for an individual depends on several factors, and decisions are best left to the physician, taking into consideration the individual's health and financial status. Drug therapy is important in osteoporotic women for whom the risk of a fracture is significantly increased. Drug therapy may also be important for reducing bone loss and preventing osteoporosis in osteopenic women at risk for developing osteoporosis. Drug therapy should never be considered a substitute for exercise, however, because of the many physical and mental wellness benefits exercise provides, including its ability to significantly reduce fall risk.

ACTION PLAN:
CONSIDERING THE PROS AND CONS OF MEDICATION

□ Know that medication may be part of your action plan for bone health if you have osteoporosis or are at significant risk for developing it.

□ Rest assured that several new osteoporosis-fighting drugs are available to help increase bone mass or prevent bone loss.

□ Have a general understanding of the available medications, including their pros and cons.

□ Work with your physician to determine whether you need medication to help manage your bone health and which medication is best for you.

□ Remember that physical activity has many benefits beyond bone health and, along with appropriate medication, may be part of an overall action plan for a healthy lifestyle.

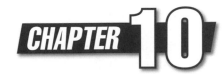

CHAPTER 10

CHARTING PROGRESS AND STAYING MOTIVATED

Although years of research have proven that regular and specific exercise can help improve and maintain your bone health and lower your risk of fracture, the science of human behavior is still trying to find the key to motivating people to exercise lifelong. It's easy for me to tell you that exercise is good for you, that there's no reason you can't exercise, and that you should do so for the rest of your life. When I was a young graduate student with a flexible schedule, no family to take care of, and the energy of youth, I didn't understand why people weren't motivated to exercise. Now that I am a full-time working professional, wife, and mother of two young children, I have a little more empathy with those who struggle to find the time and motivation to exercise. But I still exercise regularly because I have made a commitment to my health, for myself and for my family. You can do it too! In this chapter, we'll discuss strategies for fostering the motivation and commitment necessary for lifetime exercise success and for managing your program over the long term!

Ready, Set, Go!

Changing human behavior has been an incredible challenge for scientists, therapists, coaches, teachers, and individuals for centuries. An example of how difficult this challenge has been is the disappointing fact that more than one in four Americans get absolutely no leisure-time exercise at all—despite the fact that most Americans know exercise is good for them.

If you have struggled to find the motivation to exercise, you are not alone. One of the hardest steps in beginning a lifetime exercise program is making the commitment to take charge of your health. You've already shown this commitment by studying this book. Nice job! Next, you'll want to make sure you create an environment that will help foster your success as an exerciser.

Your next step should be to set goals for your program. Setting goals not only helps reinforce your commitment to yourself, but also helps you develop the framework for your program. If you don't remember the guidelines for goal setting, you might want to go back and review them in chapter 6. I suggest writing your goals on paper and posting them someplace visible—your refrigerator, your bathroom mirror, your front door—anyplace where they will be a constant reminder of your commitment to yourself. To help you do this, I've provided a sample goal-setting form on page 157. Make a copy of it or just tear it out and post it. Start making your program visible and real!

Creating Your Exercise Environment

After setting your goals, the next step is to create an environment that will foster a successful program. By *environment* I mean determining where you will exercise, who you will exercise with, what equipment you will need, and what program you will follow. If you create a favorable environment for exercise, you will set yourself up for success, and that success will be an important motivator for long-term adherence to your program.

Exercising at Home Versus in the Gym

Many people bounce back and forth between exercising at home and exercising at a health club for various reasons. When I was in my undergraduate program in California, I was interested in triathlon, so most of my training was done outdoors. Plus, the weather was reliably sunny and dry. Later in my time there, I broke my foot, so I joined a gym so I could do non-weight-bearing exercises such as swimming and stationary biking. When I moved to Oregon for graduate school, part of my student fees covered the recreation hall, so I often did my workouts in that gym. The climate was mixed there, so I spent the summer exercising outdoors and the winter exercising indoors. When I moved to Arizona for my first job, I lived in an area where it snowed half the year (yes, it was Arizona!), so I did a mix of activities, including winter sports and gym-based exercise. Now that I'm back in Oregon, working and raising a family, I don't have time to go to the gym, so I have a treadmill in our spare room and a barbell, four dumbbells, an elastic band, and an exercise ball in the closet that I break out three times a week for resistance training. When I am playing with my kids, I stretch on the floor to improve my flexibility, and we spend a lot of time jumping up and down for fun and for our bones!

When you plan your program, you will need to know whether you plan to exercise at home or someplace else. The pros and cons of exercising

▷ *Exercise Goals*

In the spaces below, write your current goals for your exercise program. Set both a short- and long-term goal. After you've been exercising regularly for a month or two, revisit your goals and modify them as you see fit. When the time you set for achieving your short-term goal arrives, reevaluate your fitness program and perhaps even retest your fitness if you did so when you started exercising, then set another short-term goal.

Post these goals in a visible place to keep you motivated.

MY SHORT-TERM EXERCISE GOAL (FOR A 3- TO 4-MONTH PERIOD)

Date: _____

Goal: _____

_____

Do I need to refine this goal? _____

Did I reach this goal? _____

Why or why not? _____

_____

MY REVISED OR NEW SHORT-TERM EXERCISE GOAL

Date: _____

Goal: _____

_____

Do I need to refine this goal? _____

Did I reach this goal? _____

Why or why not? _____

_____

MY REVISED OR NEW SHORT-TERM EXERCISE GOAL

Date: _____

Goal: _____

_____

Do I need to refine this goal? _____

Did I reach this goal? _____

Why or why not? _____

_____

MY LONG-TERM EXERCISE GOAL (THE OVERALL OBJECTIVE OF THE PROGRAM)

Date: _____

Goal: _____

_____

at home or away are summarized in table 10.1, and tips for each location are given in the sidebars on this page and on page 159. If you exercise in your house, you will need a dedicated space. If you exercise outdoors, you need a plan for what to do in inclement weather. If you exercise away from home, will you exercise at a gym, health club, or community center? How much will it cost? What are the hours? What classes are available? You may want to have a plan B for your location in case plan A doesn't work out. You don't want uncertainty about where you'll exercise to become a barrier to maintaining your program.

Table 10.1 Exercising at Home Versus at a Health Club

Location	Advantages	Disadvantages
Home	Convenient, no travel time, no membership fees, can exercise any time of day, solitude	No access to fitness professional, limited equipment options, many distractions, equipment can take up livable space, motivation can be a challenge, safety
Health club	Access to fitness professional, variety of general and specialized programs/classes and state-of-the-art equipment, motivation of group setting/social atmosphere	Transportation requirement, membership and initiation fees, environment may be intimidating for new exerciser

Tips for Exercise at Home

▸ Make sure you have adequate space and proper equipment.

▸ Make sure you can control the climate and ventilation.

▸ Make sure you have an action plan in case of an emergency or injury.

▸ Make sure you do not create an unsafe environment for others.

Exercising Alone Versus in a Group

You also need to decide whether to exercise in a group or class setting, with a partner, or alone. People tend to have strong preferences in this regard, and you should do what feels right for you. Personally, I prefer to exercise alone most of the time. I love to run, and this is my personal time away from work, family, and the commotion of everyday life. It is almost like meditation for me and is often my only time alone for the entire day. I work out my troubles, solve work problems, draft grants, smile on good

Tips for Exercise in a Health Club or Gym

▸ Health clubs do not need special licensing for operation, so you must be an informed consumer when selecting a facility.

▸ Make sure the health club is adequately staffed. Trainers should have a college degree in exercise science or a related health field or, at minimum, proper certification.*

▸ Make sure the equipment is laid out in a way that minimizes your risk of injury from tripping or falling (e.g., enough space between machines, clear walkways).

▸ If you are interested in classes, make sure they are appropriate for your initial and projected abilities. Talk to the fitness director or instructor to be sure. A good instructor should be able to accommodate various fitness levels within the same class, but this may be difficult with a mix of beginning and advanced exercisers.

▸ Make sure the climate and ventilation are adequate and, if not, that a staff member will address these issues.

▸ Make sure the environment is one in which you feel comfortable exercising. For example, if you want to start resistance training but find the weight room filled with big, bulky guys, that may not be the most welcoming environment. Find a place where you fit in with those around you. For older adults, the local YMCA or community center is often such a setting. For women, women-only health clubs may be more appealing.

*Recommended certifications: American College of Sports Medicine (ACSM), American Council on Exercise (ACE), International Dance and Education Association (IDEA)

times, or just think about nothing and notice only my surroundings. I tend to do my resistance training while watching the morning news, and I stretch on the floor with my husband and kids. I have found it hard to commit to group exercise because my schedule is so unpredictable and I hate to break commitments. I used to play more sports and enjoyed running in racing events for the camaraderie, and I look forward to taking those up again one day when my life is less hectic.

My father, on the other hand, is someone who *must* exercise with a partner or in a group to keep his motivation. Left to his own devices, he would rather work on the computer or watch soccer games on TV. My mother walks religiously every morning, and if it weren't for the fact that my father doesn't want her to walk alone, he probably wouldn't go. The women in my research studies have also preferred to exercise in a group. They enjoyed meeting new friends, and they felt a sense of obligation to show up. During class they felt challenged to keep up with the group.

When they missed a class, the others were quick to ask where they were and if everything was okay. If someone missed several classes, one of the women would usually volunteer to call her and check in.

Others find exercising in a group or gym environment somewhat intimidating. If this is the case for you, try to adjust your mind-set. You have every right to be exercising in any environment, and you should be proud to be an exerciser. To make you feel more comfortable, though, you may want to find a class or facility with clientele similar to you in age, gender, and abilities. As mentioned earlier, many women-only facilities are available, as well as gyms for adults over age 50. These facilities often provide classes more appropriate to their specific type of clients. As always, check out the facility before investing your money in a membership. Ask for a short trial period to "test drive" the facility to ensure it suits your preferences.

Obtaining Equipment

The type of equipment you need will depend on the type of exercise you choose as well as the setting in which you choose to exercise. For aerobic exercise, you may need little more than proper shoes and clothing. For resistance exercise, however, some equipment is needed to provide resistance, and more experienced exercisers may need additional equipment to progress to more challenging levels. Adding equipment might also add a new dimension to an existing program. In most cases, the necessary financial investment in equipment is minimal and should be considered justifiable, as it could save you hundreds to thousands of dollars in medical expenses by preventing or decreasing the severity of health problems.

Charting Your Progress

As you embark on your exercise program, you should keep track of how much you exercise, what you do, what you like or don't like about a particular class or workout, when you feel your best and your worst, and so on. Keeping a simple exercise log or diary is a useful tool for evaluating whether your original exercise plan is working for you and how to adjust it to better meet your needs. Some of my athlete friends like to add personal notes on their exercise logs that convey a sense of how they were feeling during and after their workout or what they liked or disliked about a particular running route, and so forth. These little notes can help you determine the conditions and the amount of exercise that are right for you. Exercise logs can also be very good motivators because you get to see your progress and your achievements on paper. One of my dearest friends, a lifelong runner, used to keep an informal running log on a piece of paper taped to his desk. He kept this log for many years, so he could see his accomplishments over time, compare one year to the next, and brag a lot! He'd keep totals of his yearly running mileage on another chart. He logged more than 15,000 miles over 20 years of running. What a testimony to his dedication to and love of running!

We've included four sample exercise logs that you can copy or use as models for your own log (see tables 10.2 through 10.5). Alternatively, you could keep notes on an oversized or personal calendar, your handheld computer, or in a journal. Some people prefer to log their exercise daily so they don't forget the specifics of their workout. Others prefer to log exercise on a weekly basis. I suggest that you log your exercise at no longer than one-week intervals because your ability to recall your workout, the environment, and your feelings about it will wane over time. No matter what medium or method you use, keeping track of your progress can motivate you to keep exercising.

You may also want to keep track of your physical and mental improvements over the course of your exercise program. In chapter 5, I described several methods for assessing your starting fitness level. By retesting yourself every three to six months, you can chart the physical improvements that are occurring in response to regular exercise. In fact, studies suggest that knowledge of physical improvements is even better motivation for continuing exercise in older adults than that provided by the social atmosphere of group exercise. The anticipation of follow-up testing was a huge motivator for the women in my exercise studies because they wanted to see the fruits of their labor. Once they realized how much they had improved, they became even more motivated to continue exercising for fear of losing their gains.

Table 10.2   Aerobic Exercise Log

Date	Activity	Intensity/pace	Time/distance	Notes
8/1/04	Alternate: walk 1 lap, jog 1 lap	HR approximately 130	12 laps on track	Felt great! Perfect weather. Listened to favorite music on iPod that energized me.

Table 10.3   Resistance Exercise Log

Date	Exercises	Weight/band color/ % body weight	Reps	Sets	Notes
8/1/04	Shoulder press	10 lb.	8	2	Feel good; leg work was hard since I ran yesterday. May increase to red band for lats.
	Chest press	20 lb.	7	2	
	Bent-over row	15 lb.	8	2	
	Lat pull-down	Green band	10	2	
	Squat	5% body weight in vest for all leg exercises	8	2	
	Front lunge		8	2	
	Side lunge		10	2	
	Heel-toe raise		10		

From *Action Plan for Osteoporosis* by Kerri Winters-Stone, © 2005 American College of Sports Medicine, Champaign, IL: Human Kinetics.

Table 10.4   Jump Exercise Log

Date	Step height or vest weight	Reps	Sets	Notes
8/1/04	4-in. step 5 lb. in vest	10	5	Just added a weighted vest. Challenging, but fun!

From *Action Plan for Osteoporosis* by Kerri Winters-Stone, © 2005 American College of Sports Medicine, Champaign, IL: Human Kinetics.

Tracking Bone Health

The main purpose of this book is to provide exercise options and plans for improving your bone health based on the most recent evidence from scientific research. This evidence is always based on the responses for a

Table 10.5   General Exercise Log

(Good for programs that include many types of exercise)				
Date	**Activity**	**Intensity**	**Duration**	**Notes**
8/1/04	Aerobics class	HR approximately 120-140	60-min class including warm-up	So-so. Tired from work.
8/2/04	Weights at gym	Most at 10RM	3 sets of 8 reps	Better day. More energy.
8/4/04	Yoga class	Don't know. I worked hard!	45-min class	Feel great. Very relaxed.

From *Action Plan for Osteoporosis* by Kerri Winters-Stone, © 2005 American College of Sports Medicine, Champaign, IL: Human Kinetics.

group of volunteers and does not guarantee that everyone will respond in the same way and to the same degree that those in the research group did. You can be reasonably assured, however, that you are following a sound, evidence-based program that will provide results.

To be absolutely sure that your bone health is responding in the expected way, you need to have a bone density test before beginning your exercise program and at least 12 months after you've been exercising regularly. Why do you need to wait so long before reassessing your bone health? As discussed earlier, bone is a dynamic but slowly adapting tissue that usually takes at least 12 months to show signs of response to a persistent challenge such as exercise.

As we age, our skeleton may need a little extra time to respond. In one of our studies, older women regularly did resistance and jump exercises for nine months and got stronger and leaner but showed little change in their bone health. After the study ended, the women wanted to continue exercising, so they clamored to have the exercises taught at the community college and local health club. Five years later, we brought these women back in and remeasured their bone density and that of the original controls. We found that the controls, who did not take part in the exercise program, lost bone at the hip at a rate of about 1 percent per year, loss that is expected due to age (Snow et al. 2000). However, the women who continued to exercise over the five years completely halted their bone loss, and some women even increased their bone density (see figure 10.1)! The message here is that it takes persistence and patience to see a measurable change in bone health. Even though you may not see a change very quickly, rest assured that these improvements will occur in time.

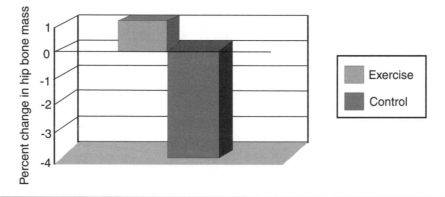

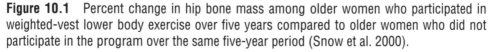

Figure 10.1 Percent change in hip bone mass among older women who participated in weighted-vest lower body exercise over five years compared to older women who did not participate in the program over the same five-year period (Snow et al. 2000).

Adapted, by permission, from C.M. Snow, J.M. Shaw, K.M. Winters, and K.A. Witzke, 2000, "Long-term exercise using weighted vests prevents hip bone loss in postmenopausal women," *J Gerontol A Biol Sci Med Sci.* 55:M489-M491. Copyright © The Gerontological Society of America. Reproduced by permission of the publisher.

In the meantime, remind yourself that you are doing the best thing you can do for your bones based on the best available evidence, and just keep plugging along. Undoubtedly, you will notice other changes sooner, such as better muscle tone, because these tissues adapt more quickly than bone. Use these changes as your motivator, along with the knowledge that you are also helping your bones! You don't necessarily need to have a follow-up bone density test to be sure you are doing the right thing. I can assure you that you are!

Staying Motivated

Finding the motivation to start a lifelong exercise program may be a challenge for you, but you have already shown your determination to take positive steps for your bone health by buying this book. I can provide you with the essential tools you need to start a safe and effective program and to keep your program working for you over time. The motivation to exercise, however, must come from within. As with any effort to change your behavior, you must do it for yourself first and for others second. Once you begin a program (and I'm confident that you will), whether exercise is completely new for you or whether you are already exercising and want to add a new element to your program, your motivation to stick with it may be challenged from time to time. In the following section, I'll describe some common barriers you might encounter in staying with your exercise routine and some strategies for overcoming them.

Addressing Barriers

Everyone encounters barriers to maintaining a regular exercise program at one time or another. Some of us face many barriers, and that makes the challenge to begin and stick with exercise even tougher. Some of the most common reasons people give for not being able to exercise or for discontinuing exercise are

- lack of time,
- lack of resources (money, location),
- lack of support from family or friends,
- unexpected or frequent travel,
- frequent or prolonged illness or injury,
- inclement weather, and
- lack of enjoyment or motivation.

Barriers can be tough to overcome but rarely impossible. Regardless of the barrier, the motivation to address and overcome it needs to come from within. That motivation comes from your internal commitment to your health. Having a few strategies at hand can help you overcome these barriers and avoid lapses in your exercise program.

Avoiding a Lapse in Your Program

In my current research, I study bone health in women with breast cancer. Most of these women are so fatigued during treatment that their activity levels inevitably fall off. But the women who were exercisers before their diagnosis are determined to resume their exercise routine when their treatment is over because they know how good exercise can make them feel.

Despite all they have been through and continue to face, they gradually and persistently regain their activity levels. These women have faced one of the ultimate barriers to exercise continuation and managed to overcome it. If they can overcome the barrier of a life-threatening illness and aggressive treatment, you, too, can overcome any barriers you face.

Occasional lapses in your exercise program are often unavoidable and not unexpected. Missing some exercise should not discourage you to the point that you give up completely, though. During a lapse, your goal should be to minimize the time that you are away from exercise and get back into your regular routine as soon as possible. Most important, don't be too hard on yourself if you do experience a lapse. Allow yourself to fall down, but dust yourself off and get right back in the saddle!

Here are some strategies for overcoming the common barriers in the previous section.

Lack of time

• *Break your exercise routine into shorter but more frequent bouts.* For example, if you are focusing on resistance exercise but can't fit a full upper and lower body workout into your day, do the upper body program on one day and the lower body program the next. Take a day of rest and then repeat upper and lower body workouts for the next two days of the week.

• *Exercise in the morning.* It sounds crazy, but I exercise between 5:00 and 5:30 in the morning. My son gets up at 6:30 a.m., and after that the day only gets more hectic. After a full day's work, I don't want to worry about exercise, so I like getting it out of the way early in the day. Morning exercise can be hard at first, but by adjusting your bedtime and sticking with it for the first few weeks, it becomes easier to do. You may even find that you enjoy the peacefulness of a morning workout.

• *Exercise on your lunch break.* Many workplaces have a gym in-house or nearby, or at least have a shower and changing area. Eat lunch at your desk or grab something quick and easy, such as a sandwich or a smoothie and an energy bar.

Lack of resources (money, location)

• *Exercise at home.* If there is no facility nearby where you can exercise, you can exercise at home. The exercise programs I've described can all be done at home with minimal equipment.

• *Exercise at a community center.* If a health club is too expensive, look for local community centers or senior centers that offer quality programs at lower cost and often provide discounts for local residents or seniors. If these are still too costly, exercise at home.

Lack of support from family or friends

• *Try to ignore negative comments.* Sometimes family members or friends are threatened by your decision to take care of yourself and to

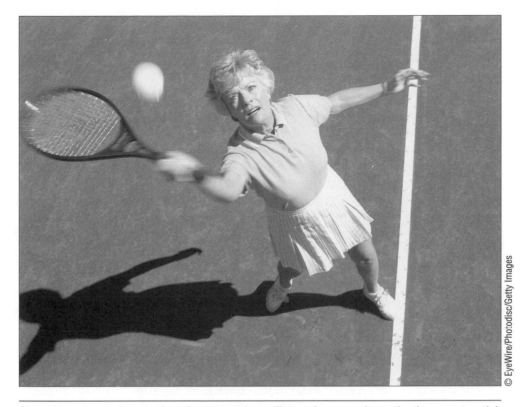

Choosing an exercise or sport that you enjoy will go a long way in motivating you to stick with it.

become active. They may be confronting their own health problems, so you may need to be tolerant of their seeming lack of support and ignore any negative criticism. Don't let anyone else sabotage the positive steps you are taking toward good health.

• *Find other support.* Exercising with people who value exercise the same way you do can be supportive and motivating. Enlist the support of exercise partners, fellow class members, and exercise leaders, and let them know that their encouragement helps you keep going.

Unexpected or frequent travel

• *Try something new.* Sometimes we must spend time away from home due to travel for work or personal reasons, including well-deserved vacations. If at all possible, take advantage of the situation and try exercising at your destination. Walking or jogging around new towns or countries can be a great way to get a feel for the area (be sure to consult with locals to find safe routes). If you are staying in a hotel, you may have several options. Most hotels have some sort of fitness center, and if not, often a local gym will let you use their facility for a daily fee. The hotel concierge can generally point you to jogging routes or other exercise areas.

- *Improvise.* No matter where you are or what kind of accommodations you have, you can usually do some sort of fitness routine in your room. Jogging or marching in place plus some easy resistance exercises using body weight (push-ups, squats, triceps dips) or bands (see chapter 7), a few balance exercises, and stretching can make for a great on-the-go routine.

- *Rest, relax, and return to exercise when you get home.* Sometimes you either can't exercise when you are traveling or just don't want to. Use this situation as a break period from exercise—a time to rest, relax, and recharge your enthusiasm for staying fit. When I am forced to take a break from exercise, I am so happy when I finally get to work out again that I find myself refreshed and ready to go. I am reminded how great exercise makes me feel, inside and out.

Frequent or prolonged illness or injury

- *Take care of yourself.* Being ill or injured can frustrate any exerciser because it causes an unforeseen break in your exercise routine. You may be tempted to exercise before you are fully recovered, but this can be a big mistake because you often end up prolonging your recovery. Trust me, I've done so and have regretted it. In the case of illness, you need to listen to your body and to your physician, if you are being treated. Once you feel better and ready to exercise, wait at least a day or two more to ensure that you don't exacerbate your illness. If you are injured, follow your physician's advice first and foremost. Give yourself ample recovery time, and remember that if you come back too early, you may have to start your recovery all over again. That can double or even triple your recovery time.

- *Be patient.* Recovery from illness or injury can take several weeks or longer, and you may become frustrated. Remind yourself that this is a temporary setback and that you are taking care of your body so that it can return to its normal routine.

- *Find alternative activities.* If you are injured, you may be able to do activities that do not aggravate the injury site. For example, when I broke my foot, I couldn't do any weight-bearing activities, but after a few weeks of inactivity, I could swim, ride the stationary bike, and lift weights with my arms. This was enough to keep me in shape until I could return to running— and kept me from being frustrated by not being able to stay active.

- *Come back slowly.* In the case of either illness or injury, return to exercise slowly and heed your body's warning signals that you may be overdoing it. If you've been injured or sick for a while, start by doing less than half your normal amount of exercise, meaning half the frequency, duration, and intensity. Over the next few weeks, gradually work your way back up to your pre-injury or pre-illness level.

Inclement weather

- *Brave the elements.* I live in Oregon, where the local seasons are some rain, rain, more rain, and a lot of rain, so I understand what a challenge weather can be for exercising outdoors. For a while I braved the weather by buying a well-insulated, wind- and waterproof running suit, hat, and shoes and going out in anything short of a severe storm. I enjoyed the solitude it gave me, because very few people were out there, and I took pride in not letting the weather keep me from staying healthy. I do this a lot less now that we have a treadmill, but I still enjoy the occasional rainy run. Braving the elements is okay as long as you are prepared to exercise in a given climate (appropriate clothes, shoes, etc.) and the conditions are not too extreme. Older adults may have a reduced ability to adapt to extremes of heat or cold, so this may be a consideration for you.

• *Enjoy seasonal activities.* Some activities or sports are only possible in certain seasons. Winter sports are a prime example and may be a great alternative to your usual routine. Although far less tested for their bone-building abilities, winter sports can help maintain your fitness and keep your exercise program fun!

• *Exercise indoors.* I must admit that, now that we have a treadmill, I prefer a dry jog over a wet one almost any day. I try to vary my treadmill run a little by adding an incline or some speed work to break up the monotony. Setting up an indoor routine or two for bad weather days is a must for anyone who lives outside of sunny California! You may also want to consider joining a gym over the bad weather season. Many health clubs offer three-month trial memberships at lower than usual rates that are perfect for these situations.

Lack of enjoyment or motivation

• *Change is good.* If you find yourself becoming bored or disinterested in your exercise program, it may be time for a change. It's not unusual for a routine to become monotonous after a while, and this is where a little creativity can help keep you interested. You don't necessarily need to adopt a whole new type of exercise; start by modifying your current routine a little. If you do aerobic exercise, try doing a different activity or adding little bursts of faster-paced work during your program, exercising outdoors instead of indoors, or taking a new class. If you do resistance exercise, substitute new exercises for old ones or try a different type of equipment (free weights instead of machines).

• *Take a break.* Perhaps your boredom is a sign that you need a vacation from exercise. Take a week or two off, but try to stay active by doing fun or interesting activities. Go dancing one evening or take a long walk at the beach or hike in a nearby park. You will likely miss your exercise routine and be ready to get back into things when you return. Don't take too much time off, though, or you will start to lose fitness that you'll have to work hard to regain.

Keeping It Fun!

Much of this chapter has focused on finding ways to stay motivated to exercise. As I mentioned at the beginning, this can be a great challenge.

As with anything you do on a regular basis, it's easier to stick to a routine if you enjoy what you are doing. You have so many types of activities to choose from that something is bound to capture your attention. You may have to try different types of exercise, different settings, different equipment, and so forth, until you find something you enjoy. You won't always like an activity at first, so be sure you give any new exercise a long enough trial run. At the same time, don't force yourself to stick with something you don't like. You will only set yourself up to get turned off by exercise in the long run. Inevitably, there will be days when it will be hard to exercise, and you may have to drag yourself to the gym. As long as it doesn't happen too often, you can usually trudge through them. On occasion, you may need to skip exercise for a day and try again the next, or you could lighten your workout for a day or two.

You're on Your Way

Clearly, you are already on your way toward adopting a positive plan for optimizing your health that includes exercising for a stronger skeleton. You've become an armchair expert on osteoporosis and how medication, diet, and particularly exercise can help lower your risk of a fracture. You now have the knowledge to develop and begin an exercise program that meets your personal needs and health goals. You have strategies to help you stay motivated and overcome barriers to sticking to your exercise program. You have all the tools you need for a lifelong program that optimizes the health of your bones. I am confident that you can and will succeed in your exercise endeavors and live a long, active, and healthy life.

ACTION PLAN:
CHARTING PROGRESS AND STAYING MOTIVATED

☐ Set short- and long-term goals for your exercise program.

☐ Understand that changes in bone health take time.

☐ Think about how you can create an exercise environment that will foster your success as an exerciser.

☐ Be aware of common barriers that might challenge your ability to stick with your exercise program.

☐ Be familiar with strategies for overcoming those barriers.

☐ Choose exercises that you enjoy, and vary your program to keep it fun.

APPENDIX: FITNESS ASSESSMENT NORMS

The following tables include norms for most of the tests in chapter 5: 1.5-mile walk or run (maximal aerobic power values), six-minute walk, two-minute step test, 1RM test (upper body and leg strength values), sit-to-stand, arm curl, sit-and-reach test, back scratch test, and up-and-go.

Table 1 *Percentile Values for Maximal Aerobic Power (mL × kg⁻¹ × min⁻¹)*

	Age				
Percentile	**20-29**	**30-39**	**40-49**	**50-59**	**60 and over**
Men					
90	51.4	50.4	48.2	45.3	42.5
80	48.2	46.8	44.1	41.0	38.1
70	46.8	44.6	41.8	38.5	35.3
60	44.2	42.4	39.9	36.7	33.6
50	42.5	41.0	38.1	35.2	31.8
40	41.0	38.9	36.7	33.8	30.2
30	39.5	37.4	35.1	32.3	28.7
20	37.1	35.4	33.0	30.2	26.5
10	34.5	32.5	30.9	28.0	23.1
Women					
90	44.2	41.0	39.5	35.2	35.2
80	41.0	38.6	36.3	32.3	31.2
70	38.1	36.7	33.8	30.9	29.4
60	36.7	34.6	32.3	29.4	27.2

(continued)

Table 1 (continued)

Percentile	Age				
	20-29	30-39	40-49	50-59	60 and over
	Women				
50	35.2	33.8	30.9	28.2	25.8
40	33.8	32.3	29.5	26.9	24.5
30	32.3	30.5	28.3	25.5	23.8
20	30.6	28.7	26.5	24.3	22.8
10	28.4	26.5	25.1	22.3	20.8

Data provided by Institute for Aerobics Research, Dallas, TX (1994). Study population for the data set was predominantly white and college educated. A modified Balke treadmill test was used with $\dot{V}O_2$max estimated from the last grade/speed achieved. The following may be used as descriptors for the percentile rankings: well above average (90), above average (70), average (50), below average (30), and well below average (10).

Adapted, by permission, from American College of Sports Medicine (ACSM), 2000, *ACSM's guidelines for exercise testing and prescription*, 6th edition (Baltimore: Lippincott Williams & Wilkins), 77.

Table 2 Six-Minute Walk Norms

Percentile rank	Age						
	60-64	65-69	70-74	75-79	80-84	85-89	90-94
	Women						
95	741	734	709	696	654	638	564
90	711	697	673	655	612	591	518
85	690	673	650	628	584	560	488
80	674	653	630	605	560	534	463
75	659	636	614	585	540	512	441
70	647	621	599	568	523	493	423
65	636	607	586	553	508	476	406
60	624	593	572	538	491	458	388
55	614	581	561	524	477	443	373
50	603	568	548	509	462	426	357
45	592	555	535	494	447	409	341
40	582	543	524	480	433	394	326
35	570	529	510	465	416	376	308

Percentile rank	Age						
	60-64	65-69	70-74	75-79	80-84	85-89	90-94
Women							
30	559	515	497	450	401	359	291
25	547	500	482	433	384	340	273
20	532	483	466	413	364	318	251
15	516	463	446	390	340	292	226
10	495	439	423	363	312	261	196
5	465	402	387	322	270	214	150
Men							
95	825	800	779	762	721	710	646
90	792	763	743	716	678	659	592
85	770	738	718	686	649	625	557
80	751	718	698	661	625	596	527
75	736	700	680	639	604	572	502
70	722	685	665	621	586	551	480
65	710	671	652	604	571	532	461
60	697	657	638	586	554	512	440
55	686	644	625	571	540	495	422
50	674	631	612	555	524	477	403
45	662	618	599	539	508	459	384
40	651	605	586	524	494	442	366
35	638	591	572	506	477	422	345
30	626	577	559	489	462	403	326
25	612	562	544	471	444	382	304
20	597	544	526	449	423	358	279
15	578	524	506	424	399	329	249
10	556	499	481	394	370	295	214
5	523	462	445	348	327	244	160

Adapted, by permission, from R.E. Rikli and C.J. Jones, 2001, *Senior fitness test manual* (Champaign, IL: Human Kinetics), 127.

Table 3   Two-Minute Step Test Norms

Percentile rank	Age						
	60-64	65-69	70-74	75-79	80-84	85-89	90-94
Women							
95	130	133	125	123	113	106	92
90	122	123	116	115	104	98	85
85	116	117	110	109	99	93	80
80	111	112	105	104	94	88	76
75	107	107	101	100	90	85	72
70	103	104	97	96	87	81	69
65	100	100	94	93	84	79	66
60	97	96	90	90	81	76	63
55	94	93	87	87	78	73	61
50	91	90	84	84	75	70	58
45	88	87	81	81	72	67	55
40	85	84	78	78	69	64	53
35	82	80	74	75	66	61	50
30	79	76	71	72	63	59	47
25	75	73	68	68	60	55	44
20	71	68	63	64	56	52	40
15	66	63	58	59	51	47	36
10	60	57	52	53	46	42	31
5	52	47	43	45	37	39	24
Men							
95	135	139	133	135	126	114	112
90	128	130	124	126	118	106	102
85	123	125	119	119	112	100	96
80	119	120	114	114	107	95	91
75	115	116	110	109	103	91	86
70	112	113	107	105	99	87	83

Percentile rank	Age						
	60-64	65-69	70-74	75-79	80-84	85-89	90-94
Men							
65	109	110	104	102	96	84	79
60	106	107	101	98	93	81	76
55	104	104	98	95	90	78	72
50	101	101	95	91	87	75	69
45	98	98	92	87	84	72	66
40	96	95	89	84	81	69	62
35	93	92	86	80	78	66	59
30	90	89	83	77	75	63	55
25	87	86	80	73	71	59	52
20	83	82	76	68	67	55	47
15	79	77	71	63	62	50	42
10	74	72	66	56	56	44	36
5	67	67	67	47	48	36	26

Adapted, by permission, from R.E. Rikli and C.J. Jones, 2001, *Senior fitness test manual* (Champaign, IL: Human Kinetics), 128.

Table 4 *Maximal Upper Body Strength*

Percentile	Age				
	20-29	30-39	40-49	50-59	60 and over
Men					
90	1.48	1.24	1.10	.97	.89
80	1.32	1.12	1.00	.90	.82
70	1.22	1.04	.93	.84	.77
60	1.14	.98	.88	.79	.72
50	1.06	.93	.84	.75	.68
40	.99	.88	.80	.71	.66
30	.93	.83	.76	.68	.63
20	.88	.78	.72	.63	.57
10	.80	.71	.65	.57	.53

(continued)

Table 4 (continued)

Percentile	Age				
	20-29	**30-39**	**40-49**	**50-59**	**60 and over**
	Women				
90	.90	.76	.71	.61	.64
80	.80	.70	.62	.55	.54
70	.74	.63	.57	.52	.51
60	.70	.60	.54	.48	.47
50	.65	.57	.52	.46	.45
40	.59	.53	.50	.44	.43
30	.56	.51	.47	.42	.40
20	.51	.47	.43	.39	.38
10	.48	.42	.38	.37	.33

Values listed represent 1RM weight in pounds pressed divided by body weight in pounds.

Data provided by the Institute for Aerobic Research, Dallas, TX (1994). Study population for the data set was predominantly white and college educated. A Universal dynamic variable resistance (DVR) machine was used to measure the 1RM. The following may be used as descriptors for the percentile rankings: well above average (90), above average (70), average (50), below average (30), and well below average (10).

Adapted, by permission, from American College of Sports Medicine (ACSM), 2000, *ACSM's guidelines for exercise testing and prescription*, 6th edition (Baltimore: Lippincott Williams & Wilkins), 82.

Table 5   Maximal Leg Strength

Percentile	Age				
	20-29	**30-39**	**40-49**	**50-59**	**60 and over**
	Men				
90	2.27	2.07	1.92	1.80	1.73
80	2.13	1.93	1.82	1.71	1.62
70	2.05	1.85	1.74	1.64	1.56
60	1.97	1.77	1.68	1.58	1.49
50	1.91	1.71	1.62	1.52	1.43
40	1.83	1.65	1.57	1.46	1.38
30	1.74	1.59	1.51	1.39	1.30

Percentile	Age				
	20-29	30-39	40-49	50-59	60 and over
Men					
20	1.63	1.52	1.44	1.32	1.25
10	1.51	1.43	1.35	1.22	1.16
Women					
90	1.82	1.61	1.48	1.37	1.32
80	1.68	1.47	1.37	1.25	1.18
70	1.58	1.39	1.29	1.17	1.13
60	1.50	1.33	1.23	1.10	1.04
50	1.44	1.27	1.18	1.05	.99
40	1.37	1.21	1.13	.99	.93
30	1.27	1.15	1.08	.95	.88
20	1.22	1.09	1.02	.88	.85
10	1.14	1.00	.94	.78	.72

Values listed represent 1RM weight in pounds pressed divided by body weight in pounds.

Data provided by the Institute for Aerobic Research, Dallas, TX (1994). Study population for the data set was predominantly white and college educated. A Universal dynamic variable resistance (DVR) machine was used to measure the 1RM. The following may be used as descriptors for the percentile rankings: well above average (90), above average (70), average (50), below average (30), and well below average (10).

Adapted, by permission, from American College of Sports Medicine (ACSM), 2000, *ACSM's guidelines for exercise testing and prescription*, 6th edition (Baltimore: Lippincott Williams & Wilkins), 77.

Table 6   Sit-to-Stand Norms

Percentile rank	Age						
	60-64	65-69	70-74	75-79	80-84	85-89	90-94
Women							
95	21	19	19	19	18	17	16
90	20	18	18	17	17	15	15
85	19	17	17	16	16	14	13
80	18	16	16	16	15	14	12

(continued)

Table 6 (continued)

Percentile rank	Age						
	60-64	65-69	70-74	75-79	80-84	85-89	90-94
Women							
75	17	16	15	15	14	13	11
70	17	15	15	14	13	12	11
65	16	15	14	14	13	12	10
60	16	14	14	13	12	11	9
55	15	14	13	13	12	11	9
50	15	14	13	12	11	10	8
45	14	13	12	12	11	10	7
40	14	13	12	12	10	9	7
35	13	12	11	11	10	9	6
30	12	12	11	11	9	8	5
25	12	11	10	10	9	8	4
20	11	11	10	9	8	7	4
15	10	10	9	9	7	6	3
10	9	9	8	8	6	5	1
5	8	8	7	6	4	4	0
Men							
95	23	23	21	21	19	19	16
90	22	21	20	20	17	17	15
85	21	20	19	18	16	16	14
80	20	19	18	18	16	15	13
75	19	18	17	17	15	14	12
70	19	18	17	16	14	13	12
65	18	17	16	16	14	13	11
60	17	16	16	15	13	12	11
55	17	16	15	15	13	12	10

Percentile rank	Age						
	60-64	65-69	70-74	75-79	80-84	85-89	90-94
Men							
50	16	15	14	14	12	11	10
45	16	15	14	13	12	11	9
40	15	14	13	13	11	10	9
35	15	13	13	12	11	9	8
30	14	13	12	12	10	9	8
25	14	12	12	11	10	8	7
20	13	11	11	10	9	7	7
15	12	11	10	10	8	6	6
10	11	9	9	8	7	5	5
5	9	8	8	7	6	4	3

Adapted, by permission, from R.E. Rikli and C.J. Jones, 2001, *Senior fitness test manual* (Champaign, IL: Human Kinetics), 125.

Table 7　Arm Curl Norms

Percentile rank	Age						
	60-64	65-69	70-74	75-79	80-84	85-89	90-94
Women							
95	24	22	22	21	20	18	17
90	22	21	20	20	18	17	16
85	21	20	19	19	17	16	15
80	20	19	18	18	16	15	14
75	19	18	17	17	16	15	13
70	18	17	17	16	15	14	13
65	18	17	16	16	15	14	12
60	17	16	16	15	14	13	12
55	17	16	15	15	14	13	11
50	16	15	14	14	13	12	11

(continued)

Table 7 (continued)

Percentile rank	Age						
	60-64	65-69	70-74	75-79	80-84	85-89	90-94
Women							
45	16	15	14	13	12	12	10
40	15	14	13	13	12	11	10
35	14	14	13	12	11	11	9
30	14	13	12	12	11	10	9
25	13	12	12	11	10	10	8
20	12	12	11	10	10	9	8
15	11	11	10	9	9	8	7
10	10	10	9	8	8	7	6
5	9	8	8	7	6	6	5
Men							
95	27	27	26	24	23	21	18
90	25	25	24	22	22	19	16
85	24	24	23	21	20	18	16
80	23	23	22	20	20	17	15
75	22	21	21	19	19	17	14
70	21	21	20	19	18	16	14
65	21	20	19	18	18	15	13
60	20	20	19	17	17	15	13
55	20	19	18	17	17	14	12
50	19	18	17	16	16	14	12
45	18	18	17	16	15	13	12
40	18	17	16	15	15	13	11
35	17	16	15	14	14	12	11
30	17	16	15	14	14	11	10
25	16	15	14	13	13	11	10

Percentile rank	Age						
	60-64	65-69	70-74	75-79	80-84	85-89	90-94
Men							
20	15	14	13	12	12	10	9
15	14	13	12	11	12	9	8
10	13	12	11	10	10	8	8
5	11	10	9	9	9	7	6

Adapted, by permission, from R.E. Rikli and C.J. Jones, 2001, *Senior fitness test manual* (Champaign, IL: Human Kinetics), 126.

Table 8 *Sit-and-Reach Test Norms*

Percentile rank	Age						
	60-64	65-69	70-74	75-79	80-84	85-89	90-94
Women							
95	8.7	7.9	7.5	7.4	6.6	6.0	4.9
90	7.2	6.6	6.1	6.1	5.2	4.6	3.4
85	6.3	5.7	5.2	5.2	4.3	3.7	2.5
80	5.5	5.0	4.5	4.4	3.6	3.0	1.7
75	4.8	4.4	3.9	3.7	3.0	2.4	1.0
70	4.2	3.9	3.3	3.2	2.4	1.8	0.4
65	3.7	3.4	2.8	2.7	1.9	1.3	-0.1
60	3.1	2.9	2.3	2.1	1.4	0.8	-0.7
55	2.6	2.5	1.9	1.7	1.0	0.4	-1.2
50	2.1	2.0	1.4	1.2	0.5	-0.1	-1.7
45	1.6	1.5	0.9	0.7	0.0	-0.6	-2.2
40	1.1	1.1	0.5	0.2	-0.4	-1.0	-2.7
35	0.5	0.6	0.0	-0.3	-0.9	-1.5	-3.3
30	0.0	0.1	-0.5	-0.8	-1.4	-2.0	-3.8
25	-0.6	-0.4	-1.1	-1.3	-2.0	-2.6	-4.4
20	-1.3	-1.0	-1.7	-2.0	-2.6	-3.2	-5.1

(continued)

Table 8 (continued)

Percentile rank	Age						
	60-64	65-69	70-74	75-79	80-84	85-89	90-94
Women							
15	-2.1	-1.7	-2.4	-2.8	-3.3	-3.9	-5.9
10	-3.0	-2.6	-3.3	-3.7	-4.2	-4.8	-6.8
5	-4.0	-3.9	-4.7	-5.0	-5.0	-6.3	-7.9
Men							
95	8.5	7.5	7.5	6.6	6.2	4.5	3.5
90	6.7	5.9	5.8	4.9	4.4	3.0	1.9
85	5.6	4.8	4.7	3.8	3.2	2.0	0.9
80	4.6	3.9	3.8	2.8	2.2	1.1	0.0
75	3.8	3.1	3.0	2.0	1.4	0.4	-0.7
70	3.1	2.4	2.4	1.3	0.6	-0.2	-1.4
65	2.5	1.8	1.8	0.7	0.0	-0.8	-1.9
60	1.8	1.1	1.1	0.1	-0.8	-1.3	-2.5
55	1.2	0.6	0.6	-0.5	-1.4	-1.9	-3.0
50	0.6	0.0	0.0	-1.1	-2.0	-2.4	-3.6
45	0.0	-0.6	-0.6	-1.7	-2.6	-2.9	-4.2
40	-0.6	-1.1	-1.2	-2.3	-3.2	-3.5	-4.7
35	-1.3	-1.8	-1.8	-2.9	-4.0	-4.0	-5.3
30	-1.9	-2.4	-2.4	-3.5	-4.6	-4.6	-5.8
25	-2.6	-3.1	-3.1	-4.2	-5.3	-5.3	-6.5
20	-3.4	-3.9	-3.9	-5.0	-6.2	-5.9	-7.2
15	-4.4	-4.8	-4.8	-6.0	-7.2	-6.8	-8.1
10	-5.5	-5.9	-5.9	-7.1	-8.4	-7.8	-9.1
5	-7.3	-7.5	-7.6	-8.8	-10.2	-9.3	-10.7

Adapted, by permission, from R.E. Rikli and C.J. Jones, 2001, *Senior fitness test manual* (Champaign, IL: Human Kinetics), 129.

Table 9   Back Scratch Test Norms

Percentile rank	Age						
	60-64	65-69	70-74	75-79	80-84	85-89	90-94
Women							
95	5.0	4.9	4.5	4.5	4.3	3.5	3.9
90	3.8	3.5	3.2	3.1	2.8	1.9	2.2
85	2.9	2.6	2.3	2.2	1.8	0.8	0.9
80	2.2	1.9	1.5	1.3	0.9	-0.1	-0.1
75	1.6	1.3	0.8	0.6	0.2	-0.9	-1.0
70	1.1	0.7	0.3	0.0	-0.4	-1.6	-1.8
65	0.7	0.2	-0.2	-0.5	-1.0	-2.1	-2.5
60	0.2	-0.3	-0.8	-1.1	-1.6	-2.8	-3.2
55	-0.2	-0.7	-1.2	-1.6	-2.1	-3.3	-3.8
50	-0.7	-1.2	-1.7	-2.1	-2.6	-3.9	-4.5
45	-1.2	-1.7	-2.2	-2.6	-3.1	-4.5	-5.2
40	-1.6	-2.1	-2.6	-3.1	-3.7	-5.0	-5.8
35	-2.1	-2.6	-3.2	-3.7	-4.2	-5.7	-6.5
30	-2.5	-3.1	-3.7	-4.2	-4.8	-6.2	-7.2
25	-3.0	-3.7	-4.2	-4.8	-5.4	-6.9	-8.0
20	-3.6	-4.3	-4.9	-5.5	-6.1	-7.7	-8.9
15	-4.3	-5.0	-5.7	-6.4	-7.0	-8.6	-9.9
10	-5.2	-5.9	-6.6	-7.3	-8.0	-9.7	-11.2
5	-6.4	-7.3	-7.9	-8.8	-9.5	-11.3	-13.0
Men							
95	4.5	3.9	3.5	2.8	3.2	1.7	0.7
90	2.7	2.2	1.8	0.9	1.2	-0.1	-1.1
85	1.6	1.0	0.6	-0.3	-0.1	-1.2	-2.2
80	0.6	0.0	-0.4	-1.3	-1.2	-2.2	-3.2

(continued)

Table 9   (continued)

Percentile rank	Age						
	60-64	65-69	70-74	75-79	80-84	85-89	90-94
Men							
75	-0.2	-0.8	-1.2	-2.2	-2.1	-3.0	-4.0
70	-0.9	-1.6	-2.0	-2.9	-2.9	-3.7	-4.7
65	-1.5	-2.2	-2.6	-3.6	-3.6	-4.3	-5.3
60	-2.2	-2.9	-3.3	-4.3	-4.3	-5.0	-6.0
55	-2.8	-3.5	-3.9	-4.9	-5.0	-5.6	-6.6
50	-3.4	-4.1	-4.5	-5.6	-5.7	-6.2	-7.2
45	-4.0	-4.7	-5.1	-6.3	-6.4	-6.8	-7.8
40	-4.6	-5.3	-5.7	-6.9	-7.1	-7.4	-8.4
35	-5.3	-6.0	-6.4	-7.6	-7.8	-8.1	-9.1
30	-5.9	-6.6	-7.0	-8.3	-8.5	-8.7	-9.7
25	-6.6	-7.4	-7.8	-9.0	-9.3	-9.4	-10.4
20	-7.4	-8.2	-8.6	-9.9	-10.2	-10.2	-11.2
15	-8.4	-9.2	-9.6	-10.9	-11.3	-11.2	-12.2
10	-9.5	-10.4	-10.8	-12.1	-12.6	-12.3	-13.3
5	-11.3	-12.1	-12.5	-14.0	-14.6	-14.1	-15.1

Adapted, by permission, from R.E. Rikli and C.J. Jones, 2001, *Senior fitness test manual* (Champaign, IL: Human Kinetics), 130.

Table 10   Up-and-Go Norms

Percentile rank	Age						
	60-64	65-69	70-74	75-79	80-84	85-89	90-94
Women							
95	3.2	3.6	3.8	4.0	4.0	4.5	5.0
90	3.7	4.1	4.0	4.3	4.4	4.7	5.3
85	4.0	4.4	4.3	4.6	4.9	5.3	6.1
80	4.2	4.6	4.7	5.0	5.4	5.8	6.7
75	4.4	4.8	4.9	5.2	5.7	6.2	7.3

Percentile rank	Age						
	60-64	65-69	70-74	75-79	80-84	85-89	90-94
Women							
70	4.6	5.0	5.2	5.5	6.1	6.6	7.7
65	4.7	5.1	5.4	5.7	6.3	6.9	8.2
60	4.9	5.3	5.6	5.9	6.7	7.3	8.6
55	5.0	5.4	5.8	6.1	6.9	7.6	9.0
50	5.2	5.6	6.0	6.3	7.2	7.9	9.4
45	5.4	5.8	6.2	6.5	7.5	8.2	9.8
40	5.5	5.9	6.4	6.7	7.8	8.5	10.2
35	5.7	6.1	6.6	6.9	8.1	8.9	10.6
30	5.8	6.2	6.8	7.1	8.3	9.2	11.1
25	6.0	6.4	7.1	7.4	8.7	9.6	11.5
20	6.2	6.6	7.3	7.6	9.0	10.0	12.1
15	6.4	6.8	7.7	8.0	9.5	10.5	12.7
10	6.7	7.1	8.0	8.3	10.0	11.1	13.5
5	7.2	7.6	8.6	8.9	10.8	12.0	14.6
Men							
95	3.0	3.1	3.2	3.3	4.0	4.0	4.3
90	3.0	3.6	3.6	3.5	4.1	4.3	4.5
85	3.3	3.9	3.9	3.9	4.5	4.5	5.1
80	3.6	4.1	4.2	4.3	4.9	5.0	5.7
75	3.8	4.3	4.4	4.6	5.2	5.5	6.2
70	4.0	4.5	4.6	4.9	5.5	5.8	6.6
65	4.2	4.6	4.8	5.2	5.7	6.2	7.0
60	4.4	4.8	5.0	5.4	6.0	6.5	7.4
55	4.5	4.9	5.1	5.7	6.2	6.9	7.7
50	4.7	5.1	5.3	5.9	6.4	7.2	8.1

(continued)

Table 10 (continued)

Percentile rank	Age						
	60-64	65-69	70-74	75-79	80-84	85-89	90-94
Men							
45	4.9	5.3	5.5	6.1	6.6	7.5	8.5
40	5.0	5.4	5.6	6.4	6.9	7.9	8.8
35	5.2	5.6	5.8	6.6	7.1	8.2	9.2
30	5.4	5.7	6.0	6.9	7.3	8.6	9.6
25	5.6	5.9	6.2	7.2	7.6	8.9	10.0
20	5.8	6.1	6.4	7.5	7.9	9.4	10.5
15	6.1	6.3	6.7	7.9	8.3	9.9	11.1
10	6.4	6.6	7.0	8.3	8.7	10.5	11.8
5	6.8	7.1	7.4	9.0	9.4	11.5	12.9

Adapted, by permission, from R.E. Rikli and C.J. Jones, 2001, *Senior fitness test manual* (Champaign, IL: Human Kinetics), 131.

REFERENCES

Adachi, J.D., S. Adami, P.D. Miller, W.P. Olszynski, D.L. Kendler, S.L. Silverman, A.A. Licata, Z. Li, and E. Gomez-Panzani. 2001. Tolerability of risedronate in postmenopausal women intolerant of alendronate. *Aging* (Milano) 13(5): 347-54.

American College of Sports Medicine (ACSM). 2005. *ACSM's guidelines for exercise testing and prescription.* 7th ed. Baltimore: Lippincott Williams & Wilkins.

American College of Sports Medicine (ACSM). 2000. *ACSM's guidelines for exercise testing and prescription.* 6th ed. Baltimore: Lippincott Williams & Wilkins.

American Geriatrics Society et al. 2001. Guideline for the prevention of falls in older persons. *Journal of the American Geriatrics Society* 49: 664-72.

Baldwin, K.M., T.P. White, S.B. Arnaud, V.R. Edgerton, W.J. Kraemer, R. Kram, D. Raab-Cullen, and C. Snow. 1996. Musculoskeletal adaptations to weightlessness and development of effective countermeasures. *Med Sci Sports Exerc* 28: 1247-53.

Bjarnason, N.H., P. Alexandersen, and C. Christiansen. 2002. Number of years since menopause: Spontaneous bone loss is dependent but response to hormone replacement therapy is independent. *Bone* 30(4): 637-42.

Black, D.M., S.R. Cummings, D.B. Karpf, J.A. Cauley, D.E. Thompson, M.C. Nevitt, D.C. Bauer, H.K. Genant, W.L. Haskell, R. Marcus, S.M. Ott, J.C. Torner, S.A. Quandt, T.F. Reiss, and K.E. Ensrud. 1996. Randomised trial of effect of alendronate on risk of fracture in women with existing vertebral fractures. Fracture Intervention Trial Research Group. *Lancet* 348(9041): 1535-41.

Cauley, J.A., L. Norton, M.E. Lippman, S. Eckert, K.A. Krueger, D.W. Purdie, J. Farrerons, A. Karasik, D. Mellstrom, K.W. Ng, J.J. Stepan, T.J. Powles, M. Morrow, A. Costa, S.L. Silfen, E.L. Walls, H. Schmitt, D.B. Muchmore, V.C. Jordan, and L.G. Ste-Marie. 2001. Continued breast cancer risk reduction in postmenopausal women treated with raloxifene: 4-year results from the MORE trial. Multiple Outcomes of Raloxifene Evaluation. *Breast Cancer Res Treat* 65(2): 125-34.

Cauley, J.A., J. Robbins, Z. Chen, S.R. Cummings, R.D. Jackson, A.Z. LaCroix, M. LeBoff, C.E. Lewis, J. McGowan, J. Neuner, M. Pettinger, M.L. Stefanick, J. Wactawski-Wende, and N.B. Watts (Women's Health Initiative investigators). 2003. Effects of estrogen plus progestin on risk of fracture and bone mineral density: The Women's Health Initiative randomized trial. *JAMA* 290(13): 1729-38.

Chesnut, C.H., 3rd, S. Silverman, K. Andriano, H. Genant, A. Gimona, S. Harris, D. Kiel, M. LeBoff, M. Maricic, P. Miller, C. Moniz, M. Peacock, P. Richardson, N. Watts, and D. Baylink. 2000. A randomized trial of nasal spray salmon calcitonin in postmenopausal women with established osteoporosis: The Prevent Recurrence of Osteoporotic Fractures Study. PROOF Study Group. *Am J Med* 109(4): 267-76.

Cumming, R.G. 1998. Epidemiology of medication-related falls and fractures in the elderly. *Drugs and Aging* 12(1): 43-53.

Cummings, S.R., D.M. Black, D.E. Thompson, W.B. Applegate, E. Barrett-Connor, T.A. Musliner, L. Palermo, R. Prineas, S.M. Rubin, J.C. Scott, T. Vogt, R. Wallace, A.J. Yates, S.S. Miller, M. Davidson, M.A. Bolognese, A.L. Mulloy, N. Heyden, M. Wu, A. Kaur, and A. Lombardi. 1998. Effect of alendronate on risk of fracture in women with low bone density but without vertebral fractures: Results from the Fracture Intervention Trial. *JAMA* 280(24): 2077-82.

Cummings, S.R., D.B. Karpf, F. Harris, H.K. Genant, K. Ensrud, A.Z. LaCroix, and D.M. Black. 2002. Improvement in spine bone density and reduction in risk of vertebral fractures during treatment with antiresorptive drugs. *Am J Med* 112(4): 281-89.

Ettinger, B., D.M. Black, B.H. Mitlak, R.K. Knickerbocker, T. Nickelsen, H.K. Genant, C. Christiansen, P.D. Delmas, J.R. Zanchetta, J. Stakkestad, C.C. Gluer, K. Krueger, F.J. Cohen, S. Eckert, K.E. Ensrud, L.V. Avioli, P. Lips, and S.R. Cummings. 1999. Reduction of vertebral fracture risk in postmenopausal women with osteoporosis treated with raloxifene: Results from a 3-year randomized clinical trial. *JAMA* 282(7): 637-45.

Fehling, P.C., L. Alekel, J. Clasey, A. Rector, and R.J. Stillman. 1995. A comparison of bone mineral densities among female athletes in impact loading and active loading sports. *Bone* 17(3): 205-10.

Fleming, K.H., and J.T. Heimbach. 1994. Consumption of calcium in the U.S.: Food sources and intake levels. *J Nutr* 124(8 Suppl): 1426S-30S.

Fuchs, R.K., J.J. Bauer, and C.M. Snow. 2001. Jumping improves hip and lumbar spine bone mass in prepubescent children: A randomized controlled trial. *J Bone Miner Res* 16(1): 148-56.

Gallagher, D., M. Visser, D. Sepulveda, et al. 1996. How useful is BMI for comparison of body fatness across age, sex and ethnic groups? *Am J Epidemiol* 143: 228-39.

Gallagher, J.C., D. Goldgar, and D. Moy. 1987. Total bone calcium in normal women: Effect of age and menopause status. *J Bone Min Res* 2(6): 491-6.

Greendale, G.A., M. Espeland, S. Slone, R. Marcus, and E. Barrett-Connor. 2002. Bone mass response to discontinuation of long-term hormone replacement therapy: Results from the Postmenopausal Estrogen/Progestin Interventions (PEPI) Safety Follow-up Study. *Arch Intern Med* 162(6): 665-72.

Greenspan, S.L., R.D. Emkey, H.G. Bone, S.R. Weiss, N.H. Bell, R.W. Downs, C. McKeever, and A.Z. LaCroix. 2002. Significant differential effects of alendronate, estrogen, or combination therapy on the rate of bone loss after discontinuation of treatment of postmenopausal osteoporosis. A randomized, double-blind, placebo-controlled trial. *Ann Intern Med* 137(11): 875-83.

Gregg, E.W., M.A. Pereira, and C.J. Caspersen. 2000. Physical activity, falls, and fractures among older adults: A review of the epidemiologic evidence. *J Am Geriatr Soc* 48(8): 883-93.

Guralnik J.M., E.M. Simonsick, L. Ferrucci, R.J. Glynn, L.F. Berkman, D.G. Blazer, P.A. Scherr, and R.B. Wallace. 1994. A short physical performance battery assessing lower extremity function: Association with self-reported disability and prediction of mortality and nursing home admission. *J Gerontol* 49(2): M85-94.

Heaney, R.P., T.M. Zizic, I. Fogelman, W.P. Olszynski, P. Geusens, C. Kasibhatla, N. Alsayed, G. Isaia, M.W. Davie, and C.H. Chesnut, 3rd. 2002. Risedronate reduces the risk of first vertebral fracture in osteoporotic women. *Osteoporos Int* 13(6): 501-5.

Hodsman, A.B., D.A. Hanley, M.P. Ettinger, M.A. Bolognese, J. Fox, A.J. Metcalfe, and R. Lindsay. 2003. Efficacy and safety of human parathyroid hormone-(1-84) in increasing bone mineral density in postmenopausal osteoporosis. *J Clin Endocrinol Metab* 88(11): 5212-20.

Hoeger, W.W.K., S.L. Barette, D.R. Hale, et al. 1987. Relationship between repetitions and selected percentages of one repetition maximum. *J Appl Sport Sci Res* 1: 11-13.

Hoeger, W.W.K., and S.A. Hoeger. 1998. *Lifetime Physical Fitness and Wellness.* Englewood, CO: Morton Publishing.

Horber, F.F., S.A. Kohler, K. Lippuner, and P. Jaeger. 1996. Effect of regular physical training on age-associated alteration of body composition in men. *Eur J Clin Invest* 26(4): 279-85.

Hornbrook, M.C., V.J. Stevens, D.J. Wingfield, J.F. Hollis, M.R. Greenlick, and M.G. Ory. 1994. Preventing falls among community-dwelling older persons: Results from a randomized trial. *Gerontologist* 34(1): 16-23.

Hui, S.L., L. Zhou, R. Evans, C.W. Slemenda, M. Peacock, C.M. Weaver, C. McClintock, and C.C. Johnston, Jr. 1999. Rates of growth and loss of bone mineral in the spine and femoral neck in white females. *Osteoporosis Int* 9: 200-5.

Institute of Medicine Food and Nutrition Board. 1997. *Dietary Reference Intakes for Calcium, Phosphorus, Magnesium, Vitamin D, and Fluoride.* Washington, D.C.: National Academy Press.

Knopp, R.H., X. Zhu, and B. Bonet. 1994. Effects of estrogens on lipoprotein metabolism and cardiovascular disease in women. *Atherosclerosis* 110(Suppl): S83-91.

Kohrt, W.M., S.A. Bloomfield, K.D. Little, M.E. Nelson, and V.R. Yingling. 2004. ACSM Position Stand on Physical Activity and Bone Health. *Med Sci Sports Exerc* 36(11): 1985-96.

Leonetti, H.B., S. Longo, and J.N. Anasti. 1999. Transdermal progesterone cream for vasomotor symptoms and postmenopausal bone loss. *Obstet Gynecol* 94(2): 225-28.

Lohman, T.G. 1982. Use of body composition methodology in sports medicine. *The Physician and Sports Med* 10: 46-58.

Looker, A.C., E.S. Orwoll, et al. 1997. Prevalence of low femoral bone density in older U.S. adults from NHANES III. *J Bone Miner Res* 12(11): 1761-8.

McKay, H.A., M.A. Petit, R.W. Schutz, J.C. Prior, S.I. Barr, and K.M. Khan. 2000. Augmented trochanteric bone mineral density after modified physical education classes: A randomized school-based exercise intervention study in prepubescent and early pubescent children. *J Pediatr* 136(2): 156-62.

Michaelsson, K., H. Lithell, B. Vessby, and H. Melhus. 2003. Serum retinol levels and the risk of fracture. *N Engl J Med* 348(4): 287-94.

National Osteoporosis Foundation. 2004. Disease Statistics [Online]. Available: http://www.nof.org.

Pate, R.R., M. Pratt, S.N. Blair, W.L. Haskell, C.A. Macera, C. Bouchard, D. Buchner, W. Ettinger, G.W. Heath, A.C. King, et al. 1995. Physical activity and public health. A recommendation from the Centers for Disease Control and Prevention and the American College of Sports Medicine. *JAMA* 273: 402-07.

Pfeifer, M., M. Sinaki, P. Geusens, S. Boonen, E. Preisinger, and H.W. Minne. 2004. Musculoskeletal rehabilitation in osteoporosis: A review. *J Bone Miner Res* (8): 1208-14.

Ray, W., and M.R. Griffin. 1990. Prescribed medications and the risk of falling. *Topics in Geriatric Rehabilitation* 5: 12-20.

Riggs, B.L. 2002. Endocrine causes of age-related bone loss and osteoporosis. *Novartis Found Symp* 242: 247-59; discussion 260-64.

Riggs, B.L., H.W. Wahner, L.J. Melton, L.S. Richelson, H.L. Judd, and K.P. Offord. 1986. Rates of bone loss in appendicular and axial skeletons of women: Evidence of substantial vertebral bone loss before menopause. *J Clin Invest* 77: 1487-91.

Rikli, R.E., and C.J. Jones. 2001. *Senior Fitness Test Manual* (pp. 25-79). Champaign, IL: Human Kinetics.

Robinson, T.L., C. Snow-Harter, D.R. Taaffe, D. Gillis, J. Shaw, and R. Marcus. 1995. Gymnasts exhibit higher bone mass than runners despite similar prevalence of amenorrhea and oligomenorrhea. *J Bone Miner Res* 10(1): 26-35.

Sherrington, C., S.R. Lord, and C.F. Finch. 2004. Physical activity interventions to prevent falls among older people: Update of the evidence. *J Sci Med Sport* 7(1 Suppl): 43-51.

Snow, C.M, J.M. Shaw, K.M. Winters, and K.A. Witzke. 2000. Long-term exercise using weighted vests prevents hip bone loss in postmenopausal women. *J Gerontol* 55: M489-91.

Tinetti, M.E., and M. Speechley. 1989. Prevention of falls among the elderly. *N Engl J Med* 320(16): 1055-59.

Tinetti, M.E., and C.S. Williams. 1997. Falls, injuries due to falls, and the risk of admission to a nursing home. *N Engl J Med* 337(18): 1279-84.

Tonino, R.P., P.J. Meunier, R. Emkey, J.A. Rodriguez-Portales, C.J. Menkes, R.D. Wasnich, H.G. Bone, A.C. Santora, M. Wu, R. Desai, and P.D. Ross. 2000. Skeletal benefits of alendronate: 7-year treatment of postmenopausal osteoporotic women. Phase III Osteoporosis Treatment Study Group. *J Clin Endocrinol Metab* 85(9): 3109-15.

U.S. Department of Health and Human Services. 2004. *Bone Health and Osteoporosis: A Report of the Surgeon General* [Online]. Available: http://www.surgeongeneral.gov/library/bonehealth/.

Wassertheil-Smoller, S., S.L. Hendrix, M. Limacher, G. Heiss, C. Kooperberg, A. Baird, T. Kotchen, J.D. Curb, H. Black, J.E. Rossouw, A. Aragaki, M. Safford, E. Stein, S. Laowattana, and W.J. Mysiw (Women's Health Initiative investigators). 2003. Effect of estrogen plus progestin on stroke in postmenopausal women: The Women's Health Initiative: A randomized trial. *JAMA* 289(20): 2673-84.

Winters, K.M., and C.M. Snow. 2000. Detraining reverses positive effects of exercise on the musculoskeletal system in premenopausal women. *J Bone Miner Res* 15: 2495-2503.

Winters, K. M., and C. Snow. 2003. Initial values predict musculoskeletal response to exercise in premenopausal women. *Med Sci Sports Exerc* 35(10): 1691-96.

Wolf, S., H. Barnhart, N. Kutner, E. McNeely, C. Coogler, and T. Xu. 1996. Reducing frailty and falls in older persons: An investigation of tai chi and computerized balance training. Atlanta FICSIT Group. Frailty and Injuries: Cooperative Studies of Intervention Techniques. *J Am Geriatr Soc* 44: 489-97.

Wolff, I., J.J. van Croonenborg, H.C. Kemper, P.J. Kostense, and J.W. Twisk. 1999. The effect of exercise training programs on bone mass: A meta-analysis of published controlled trials in pre- and postmenopausal women. *Osteoporos Int* 9(1): 1-12.

Zingmond, D.S., L.J. Melton, and S.L. Silverman. 2004. Increasing hip fracture incidence in California Hispanics, 1983 to 2000. *Osteoporos Int* 15(8): 603-10.

INDEX

Note: The italicized *f* and *t* following page numbers refer to figures and tables, respectively.

ABOUT THE AUTHOR

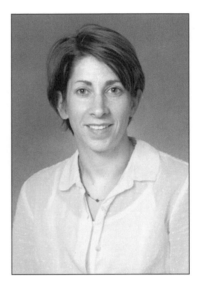

Kerri Winters-Stone is an exercise physiologist who has conducted research in the field of bone health and osteoporosis for more than a decade. She has aided in the development of exercise programs that improve bone health and reduce fall risk in adults, including the elderly, and she has obtained funding, including a grant from NASA, to develop and test exercise programs to reduce fracture risk in a variety of populations.

Winters-Stone earned her PhD in human performance from Oregon State University and her master's degree in exercise science from the University of California at Davis. Her research has been published in various outlets and presented at scientific meetings in both academic and community class settings. She is a member of the American College of Sports Medicine (ACSM), the American Society of Bone and Mineral Research, and the Oregon Gerontological Association.

Winters-Stone resides in Portland, Oregon, with her husband and their two young sons, where she remains active through running, weight training, and hiking.

ABOUT THE ACSM

The **American College of Sports Medicine (ACSM)** is an association of more than 20,000 international, national, and regional chapter members in 80 countries. It is internationally known as the leading source of state-of-the-art research and information on sports medicine and exercise science. Learn about health and fitness, nutrition, sport-specific training and injuries, and more on the ACSM Web site: www.acsm.org.

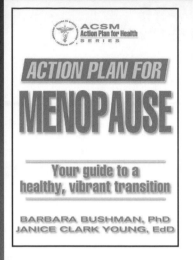
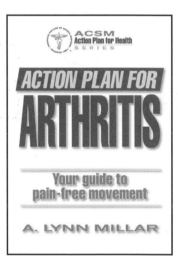
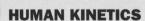